Estrogen Versus Cancer

ESTROGEN VERSUS CANCER

ZSUZSANNA SUBA

Nova Biomedical Books
New York

For permission to use material from this book please contact us:
Telephone 631-231-7269; Fax 631-231-8175
Web Site: http://www.novapublishers.com

Library of Congress Cataloging-in-Publication Data

Suba, Zsuzsanna.
Estrogen versus cancer / Zsuzanna Suba.
p. ; cm.
Includes bibliographical references and index.
ISBN 978-1-60456-949-0 (hardcover)
1. Mouth--Cancer--Endocrine aspects. 2. Mouth--Cancer--Risk factors. 3. Mouth--Cancer--Etiology. 4. Estrogen--Physiological effect. I. Title.
[DNLM: 1. Mouth Neoplasms--etiology. 2. Estrogens--deficiency. 3. Risk Factors. WU 280 S941e 2009]
RC280.M6.S83 2009
616.99'431--dc22

2008041204

Published by Nova Science Publishers, Inc. ✢ New York

Contents

Preface

Oral Cancer is a neoplasm with a fairly large male to female ration in most populations. Moreover, it develops in older age in females in comparison with males, and the ration of non-smokers, non-drinkers among elderly female oral cnacer cases if suprisingly high. The conspicuously lower incidence of this tumor among women than men is suggestive of certain endocrine involvement in its development. There are no available literary data as yet which would give an explantion to this gender specific incidence of oral cancer.

Oral cancer is a multicasual disease and there are thorough interrelationships among the etiologic factors. Till now, exogenous harmful noxae (tobacco, alcohol comsumption and energy rich diet) were overemphasized in its epidemology. However, these exogenous factors have not only local carcinogenic effect in the oral cavity, but also induce systemtic changes by means of metabolic and hormonal pathways. With full knowledge of these correlations, isolated investigations of exogenous risk factors may be misleading. This book containing the author's results on oral cancer raises a new concept concerning tumor initiation. Not estrogen, but its deficiency may provoke malignant transformation. This new theory may explain many controversial literary data concerning the associations of female sexual steroids and maliginancies.

Prologue: The Beginning

This work is a history of recognition of the anticancer capacity of the female sexual steroid, estrogen.

The first challenge was the mystery of smoking associated cancers without smoking. Accumulation of non-smoker, non-drinker elderly females among smoking associated oral cancer cases raised the plausible idea: their common feature is the postmenopausal state. How can we find an explanation for the correlation between oral cancer and postmenopausal state? Establishment that estrogen deficiency is a cancer risk factor may be the correct answer.

The further steps followed like an avalanche. The extremely rare cases of young women with oral cancer regularly exhibited hormonal disorders, such as irregular menstrual cycles, infertility or polycystic ovarium syndrome. Furthermore, in the history of middle aged female oral cancer cases a primary ovarian failure or complete hysterectomy was a conspicuously frequent finding suggestive of an estrogen deficient milieu.

There were many striking contradictions concerning the associations of female sexual steroids and cancer risk as well. Till now, breast and endometrial cancers were regarded as typically estrogen-induced tumors, particularly in postmenopausal cases. However, recent clinical studies on postmenopausal women with hormone substitution yielded unexpected and fairly controversial associations with malignancies. Unexplained, beneficial anticancer effects of hormone replacement therapy were reported against cancers at several sites, even tumors of the highly hormone sensitive organs. Re-evaluation of the results of earlier studies, which endeavored to justify the carcinogenic capacity of estrogen, exhibited many shortcomings and controversies.

Finally, the new findings both on smoking associated and hormone related tumors added up to the same conversion; not estrogen but rather its deficiency might provoke cancer initiation.

Thorough review of the literary data justified that the exquisite regulatory capacity of estrogen and its surveillance on growth, development, differentiation and metabolism are indispensable, whereas an estrogen deficient milieu may induce a breakdown in gene regulation. Nevertheless, a carcinogenic capacity of estrogen would be a failure of Nature.

This new theory of estrogen deficiency-induced carcinogenesis proves to be a philosophers' stone and supplies solution for many exiting questions in medicine. It may clarify the fairly controversial clinical and experimental associations between female sexual steroids and malignancies and justify the role of estrogen in female longevity.

Estrogen deficiency as a cancer risk factor may bring about revolutionary changes in the majority of medical disciplines: in internal medicine, endocrinology, surgery, gynecology and oncology and may provide new insight into the etiology of malignancies.

Chapter 1

Global Trends in Oral Cancer Epidemiology in the XXth Century

Dethronement of Tobacco

In recent years epidemiology has played an increasingly important role in the determination of factors that influence the development of cancer in man. The ultimate goal of these studies is to establish routes by means of which a given disease can be avoided. In searching for etiological factors one should study all possible genetic and environmental factors in order to determine the relationship of any of these players to the disease process. The incidence pattern of cancers and the trends of their morbidity and mortality over time may serve as pivotal clues to find defensive measures.

Nowadays, oral cancer is the 6th leading cause of cancer related mortality in the economically developed countries [37]. The significance of oral squamous cell cancer as a public health problem is great as it has a very high mortality rate in spite of the modern therapeutic possibilities [11]. Prevention and early diagnosis of oral cancer are extremely important to reduce the death rate.

Traditional Risk Factors for Oral Cancer

Smoking and alcohol are at the forefront on the traditional list of etiologic factors for oral cancer [4,15,33,35,37,46]. The majority of the literary data states categorically that tobacco has been well established as a leading risk factor for oral cancer [23,26,37,69,80]. Epidemiological studies have shown strong correlations between intensity and period of tobacco exposure and oral cancer risk [32]. Approximately two thirds of oral cancer cases have been attributed to traditional risk factors such as tobacco and alcohol [15,33,35,37,46,68]. Earlier, oral cancer was typically associated with men aged 60 years and older with regular tobacco and alcohol consumption, but nowadays the demography of the patients is changing [49].

Recently, controversial epidemiological data have emerged in some populations. In Greece excessive tobacco use of the male population is associated with conspicuously low morbidity and mortality of oral cancer [16]. The well-known Greek paradoxon suggests that favorable lifestyle and dietary habits may compensate the carcinogenic potential of tobacco.

Ethanol in itself has no carcinogenic potential, however oral microorganisms in the neglected mouth may metabolize it [67]. Metabolic products, such as acetaldehyde, may have strong toxic and carcinogenic impact [29].

The role of alcohol consumption alone in the development of oral cancer may be hardly assessed as it overlaps with other possible etiological agents, especially with tobacco. Tobacco and alcohol have a strong synergism in their cancer provoking effect as together they increase the mucosal permeability for carcinogenic compounds [37]. Many authors concluded that the combined risk for oral cancer is greater than the additive effect and seems to be multiplicative [20,22,49]. In the United States case-control studies justified that alcohol and tobacco potentiate each other and this common effect results in multiplication of the cancer risk [32].

Dietary habits have important role in the maintenance of oral health. A Mediterranean diet predominantly implying vegetables, fruits, olive oil and unsaturated fats, is regarded as a low risk factor for oral and pharyngeal cancers [21,22,27,44,54,72,88,91]. On the contrary, diets with excessive intake of saturated fatty acids or sweets with high glycemic index are strongly associated with cancer risk at several sites. Correlations between diet, metabolic state and oral cancer are discussed in detailed in Chapter 2.

Clinical and epidemiological studies justified that *neglected oral hygiene*, defective or lost teeth, periodontal inflammation, as well as low frequency of dental check-ups emerged as strong risk factors for oral cancer [48]. However, regular dental check-ups were associated with decreased oral cancer risk [71]. Nowadays, plaque induced chronic periodontitis is also regarded as risk for oral cancer [82].

Recently, the *role of viruses* in the development of oral cancer has received great interest, and particular attention has been paid to the human papilloma virus [13]. Some subtypes of this virus may be found in oropharyngeal tumors and they increase the incidence of oral cancer [25,58]. However, the incidence of HPV-related oral cancer is relatively low, making the association between HPV and oral malignancies unclear as yet.

Genetic factors may have important role in oral cancer inclination [87]. Deletion of tumor suppressor genes at certain chromosomal regions is closely associated to squamous cell cancers of the head and neck [18,52]. Polymorphisms in nucleotide excision repair genes may contribute to genetic susceptibility to oral leukoplakia and may contribute to the development of oral cancer [86]. It is a very great problem to discern whether raised risk for oral cancer may be determined by an interaction between inherent genetic susceptibility and exposure to carcinogens, or by unhealthy habits alone [50,51].

Studies on non-smoker oral cancer cases clarified that there are differences in the chromosomal changes between smoker and non-smoker oral cancer patients [38]. These data suggest that individual genetic inclination may also have a decisive role in the carcinogenic effect of tobacco and alcohol [29].

Immune deficiency is a well-known risk factor for all cancer types. Increased incidence of malignancies has been documented in chronic immunodeficiency states disregarding their origin [76]. Oral cancer has been reported in patients undergoing immunosuppressive therapy following organ transplantation [85]. Cell mediated immunity is also unfavorably affected by betel quid chewing, which is a high risk factor for oral cancer in India [9]. Otherwise, individuals with increased immunoreactivity and allergic diseases have decreased risk for cancers of the oral cavity and several other sites [57].

Other Factors Affecting the Epidemiology of Oral Cancer

There are striking differences in the incidence and prevalence of oral cancer among inhabitants of different *geographic regions*.

In some parts of India oral cancer accounts for approximately 35% of all cancers. In Asian populations betel-quid chewing with or without the inclusion of tobacco has long been identified as a major risk factor for oral cancer [49]. Fifty percent of oral cancers in India occur in the buccal mucosa in contrast to a less than 5% in many western countries [73]. This high-risk location is associated with the harmful effect of tobacco and betel-quid chewing [4].

On the contrary, in the United States oral cancer incidence is much lower. The estimated newly diagnosed oral cancer cases account for 3% of all malignancies in men and 2% in women [11,66].

In Europe the Mediterranean countries (Greece, Albania, Jugoslavia) show conspicuously lower oral cancer morbidity as compared with the countries in a continental position (Hungary, Slovakia, Czech Republic), which seems to be independent of their socioeconomic development. This may be partially explained by the different dietary habits and lifestyle of the inhabitants [16].

A gender related high oral cancer risk for female cases was observed in the northern countries already in the 50s of the past century. In Swedish women a consistently higher prevalence of oral cancer was registered as compared with that of women in America and in other southern countries [90]. In recent studies a separate analysis of the data of male and female patients in Europe revealed also an increased all cancer morbidity and mortality among women as compared with men in the northern countries (Denmark, Iceland, Norway and Sweden) but not among men [64]. These observations suggest a gender related carcinogenic capacity of the long lasting darkness in northern countries. On the contrary, in the southern Mediterranean regions longer summer and daylight exposition may at least partially explain the lower cancer morbidity and mortality rates.

There are contradictory data concerning the correlations of *long lasting darkness* and cancer. As all cancer incidence favors for women in the northern countries, a gender related unfavorable hormonal and metabolic effect of darkness may be supposed.

The pineal hormone melatonin is the mediator of light to the physiological adaptation to day and night rhythm of humans and animals [70]. Shortage of light and sunshine in the long winter of northern regions may provoke excessive melatonin synthesis in the pineal gland, which has thorough effects by means of metabolic and hormonal pathways. There are literary data to support that in female night shift workers an increased breast cancer risk can be observed [5]. As the artificial light used at night is scarcely comparable with daylight and night shift workers sleep daytime, these female workers may have a severe lack of light exposure and increased melatonin level. In animal experiments melatonin promoted the growth of B16 melanoma [60].

Table 1.1. Cancer mortality data between 1975 and 2001 in Hungary

Year	Lung		Colorect.		Stomach		Oral cavity		Breast	Testis	Melanoma		All		
	Male	Female	Male	Female	Male	Female	Male	Female	Female	Male	Male	Female	Male	Female	Together
1975	3414	755	1477	1548	2558	1740	383	79	1674	58	86	82	13738	11776	25514
1977	3676	809	1553	1676	2526	1680	424	90	1704	85	72	90	14126	11822	25948
1979	4158	878	1655	1723	2422	1579	487	106	1802	59	91	103	14954	11991	26945
1981	4397	963	1817	1857	2277	1483	615	108	1872	56	142	108	15467	12422	27889
1983	4600	1089	1837	1896	2069	1391	668	112	1840	67	113	116	15773	12644	28417
1985	4721	1115	1889	1967	1854	1275	719	135	1999	76	117	105	15857	12671	28528
1987	5224	1302	2200	2047	1767	1210	819	166	2119	73	152	152	16626	13206	29832
1989	5145	1397	2163	2024	1745	1204	935	163	2112	76	142	131	17123	13323	30446
1991	5487	1520	2191	2272	1703	1141	1064	166	2178	73	177	143	17872	13535	31407
1993	5703	1733	2239	2182	1596	1119	1200	221	2310	49	156	137	18072	14129	32201
1995	5728	1823	2350	2254	1486	1102	1223	196	2239	53	162	145	18525	14416	32941
1997	5816	1947	2554	2229	1344	1030	1314	215	2323	40	157	156	18986	14472	33458
1999	5797	2086	2598	2314	1354	952	1361	257	2356	49	157	158	19030	14791	33821
2001	5741	2161	2594	2258	1316	850	1432	305	2304	47	188	137	18807	14511	33318

A further interesting association is the formation of estrogenic products from environmental phthalate esters under light exposure, which may also be involved in estrogen receptor mediated impacts of daylight [63]. Associations of darkness and preferential cancer risk among women seem to be possible but require further thorough investigations.

In the USA oral cancer prevalence was fairly determined by the *racial differences* of the patients. Decreasing death rates due to oral cancer were registered among pooled white males; however, rising trends in the incidence and mortality of tongue cancer among young black males have been reported [10,14]. The distribution of oral squamous cell carcinoma between black and white South Africans was also examined [19]. It was reported that the disease was more prevalent among black patients under the age of 50 when compared with whites in the same age group.

The correlation between *socioeconomic status* and cancer mortality is well known [6,39]. The example of two neighboring countries, Austria and Hungary justifies well this association [16]. Historically and geographically these countries have a lot in common and are similar in many aspects. However, since the 2nd World War they have been situated in opposite political blocks. Until the late 1960s the overall cancer mortality was quite similar in these countries, but by the early 1970s cancer mortality rates markedly declined in Austria, whereas showed a steadily increasing rate in Hungary.

In the United States the mortality rate from oral cancer varies with the socioeconomic differences of patients. Unfortunately, African-Americans tend to present with more advanced oral cancer and more ominously, their survival is lower at each stage as compared with Caucasian cases [11]. These racial differences are closely associated with the disadvantageous socioeconomic status.

In Hungary a stomato-oncological screening study among homeless people justified that precancerous lesions and oral cancer are more frequent in this group as compared with the general population [81].

Controversial Changes in Oral Cancer Epidemiology

There are temporary *changes in the morbidity and mortality of* oral cancer. In most European countries oral cancer mortality for men had been rising appreciably till the late 1980s, and also for women whose rates were markedly lower though some steady upward trend was observed [43]. In oral cancer mortality until the early 1990s upward trends were registered also in the USA and India [28,74].

A favorable decrease in alcohol and tobacco consumption in the developed European countries resulted in a declining trend in oral cancer morbidity and mortality from the 90s [45]. However, persisting rises of oral cancer morbidity and mortality were registered for most central and eastern European countries till the early 2000s, reaching exceedingly high rates in Hungary, Slovakia, Slovenia and the Russian Federation [16,43]. Prominent Hungarian demographers talked about a “health crisis east of the river Elbe” [36].

Steeply increasing ratios of oral cancer mortality both among male and female cases in the majority of central European countries and especially in Hungary are usually attributed to the excessive smoking and alcohol consumption habits [32,43]. However, the rates of these bad habits show a 15-16% difference between the Hungarian male and female population, which could hardly justify a four- to six-fold excess of male patients among oral cancer cases [78].

After some years of decline both the incidence and mortality of oral cancer in the developed countries have been raising again at the end of the century just ended, despite the fairly decreased ratio of smokers and drinkers [49].

Recently, a continuously increasing prevalence of *non-smoker non-drinker patients* is also conspicuous among oral cancer cases, especially among women [49,74,75]. This trend suggests that the decreasing incidence of smoking and drinking contributes to the appearance of earlier unknown, hidden risk factors for oral cancer.

Changes in *alcohol and tobacco use* in the examined populations are crucial as these bad habits are regarded as the major risk factors for oral and pharyngeal cancers [2]. However, a long period may elapse between the onset of exposure to a carcinogenic agent and the clinical manifestation of cancer. Development of smoking associated cancer can take upwards of 15-20 years. The prevailing smoking habits of 15-20 years ago are dominantly influencing the current mortality rate [16].

In the United States the *high male to female ratio* of oral cancer occurrence has declined continuously; from 10:1 in 1930 to 6:1 in 1950 to almost 2:1 today [11]. Similar observations have been reported in European countries. The Hungarian epidemiological data also support a declining tendency of the male to female ratio of oral cancer incidence in the past two decades from 5.8:1 to 3.7:1 [78]. These data suggested more increased tobacco and alcohol consumption among women as compared with men but such data concerning the tumor free control population were not justified.

Geographic and temporary changes in the *prevalent sites* of oral cancer also supply important clues to study the effect of tumor provoking factors. In most populations the prevalence of lower lip cancer is decreasing and that of sublingual cancer is increasing [11]. The first observation may be at least partially explained by the wide spread use of filtered cigarettes and the decreased exposition to ultraviolet irradiation as occupational injury. Spread of information concerning the dangers of excessive sunbathing and solarium use is also benevolent. In the United States lip cancer was more common in the southern states with a longer exposure to sunlight, whereas other intraoral cancer locations occurred in a fairly uniform pattern [90]. The increasing prevalence of sublingual cancers suggests an enhanced exposition to exogenous harmful chemicals, as these are dissolved in the saliva and accumulated in the horseshoe of the floor of the mouth to exert a direct carcinogenic effect.

The oral cancer *incidence among younger adults* is also increasing in many European and high incidence countries [49]. Studies from the UK and Scotland have reported rising trends of oral cancer particularly for the tongue among young cases [31,53]. Statistical analysis in the USA provided evidence for an increased prevalence of tongue cancer cases that occurred in adults younger than 40 years, from 3% in 1973 to approximately 6% in 1993 [59]. This rising oral cancer incidence in the population under 40 is also reflected in India, where 16-28% of all oral cancer patients seen at various institutions were young [65].

Surprisingly, the epidemiological features of oral cancer in young age (under 40 yrs) are quite different as compared with older cases. The younger the mean age of the examined group of oral cancer patients the lower the excess of male patients [30,50]. A case control study on oral cancer cases less than 45 years of age in south England established near equal incidence of male and female patients [51]. Even a higher frequency of oral cancer in young women than young men was reported in contrast with the sex distribution observed in older patients [41].

In a study from Japan the male to female ratio of oral cancer is considered to increase continuously with age, leading to a much higher incidence rate overall in males than in females [83]. In Hungary, our case control study resulted in somewhat different data. Above 60 years of age an increasing prevalence of female cases was demonstrated among oral cancer patients. This trend resulted in a continuous decline of the male to female ratio in this elderly population with oral cancer (see Chapter 5).

The substantial number of young cases without any known risk factors, particularly among females, reveals that factors other than tobacco and alcohol exposure may be implicated in the development of oral cancer in this age group [49]. Moreover, exposure to carcinogens such as alcohol and tobacco might be of too short duration for malignant transformation to occur in young patients [7,34]. In a high proportion of young female oral cancer cases no apparent risk factors could be found [8,55,83]. Similarly, none of the usual risk factors such as smoking, excessive drinking or poor oral hygiene were found in patients under 30 with carcinoma of the tongue [7,62].

The predominant location of oral cancer is also different in younger and older patient groups. While in unselected patient groups the floor of mouth is the prevailing tumor location, tongue cancer has a primacy among the young cases, either males or females [30,49].

Considering the literary data there is no consensus as to whether oral cancer in the young is a distinct entity from that of older cases [1,12,41] or whether the risk factors are similar as for older patients [8,47]. This work will support the latter opinion as our recent studies have revealed that systemic, hormonal and metabolic alterations strongly affect the incidence rate of oral cancer (see Chapters 3, 5 and 8). Moreover, it is to be underlined that effects of many risk factors, included tobacco and alcohol may converge to a common pathway to promote malignant transformation.

Oral Cancer: Morbus Hungaricus in the XXIst Century

Epidemiological studies on cancer mortality justify that Europe is divided into two parts by the rate of cancer deaths. Overall cancer mortality in Europe shows a decreasing trend since the early 1990s due to the widespread preventive measures. However, in the central and eastern European countries all cancer mortality has actually continued to increase [16]. These severe differences may be explained by variable lifestyle and environmental exposure, which are inevitably linked to political, social and economic inequalities.

Patterns of cancer mortality for all tumor types are very different in the European countries. Hungary is marching at the head and other post-communistic countries, like Croatia, Czech Republic, Slovakia and Poland, are close by, especially regarding the male cases. However, in the southern Mediterranean countries, such as; Bulgaria and Albania the mortality for several cancer types is conspicuously low, whereas their socioeconomic situation is quite similar or even worse as compared with the central European countries.

Hungary is the leader both in oral cancer morbidity and mortality among the European countries [64] and their steeply increasing trends are also shocking. In 1948 mortality rate for oral cancer was 2.7/100 000 persons, whereas in 2004 it was 16.7/100 000, which reflects a 6-fold increase [17]. Oral cancer mortality increased also dramatically in Hungary between 1975 and 2002, to near fourfold both among the male and female populations (374% and 386%, respectively) [24]. These disastrous epidemiological findings in Hungary are also debated among epidemiologists of the western countries and are essentially interpreted as severe exposure to tobacco and alcohol [43,45].

Epidemiological Changes of Oral Cancer Incidence over a 20-Year Calendar Period in Hungary

During a given period temporary changes in male to female oral cancer ratio, in gender related intraoral tumor sites and in exposure to the major risk factors among men and women are crucial informations.

Over a period between 1 January 1985 and 31 December 2005, oral cancer cases and tumor-free controls were studied in two phases in the Department of Oral and Maxillofacial Surgery of the Semmelweis University [78]. Patients with squamous cell oral cancer were diagnosed and treated in the Department. Control cases were complaint-free adults who volunteered to participate in a stomato-oncological screening in the same period. The mean age of the control male and female patients was chosen so as to be within one year of the mean age of the male and female oral cancer cases.

In the 1st phase of the study, between 1 January 1985 and 31 December 1986, 460 cases with histologically confirmed oral squamous cell cancer and 350 tumor-free control cases were included. In the 2nd phase of the study, between 1 January 2004 and 31 December 2005, the data of 550 oral cancer cases and 450 tumor-free controls were examined.

Male to female ratios of oral cancer cases were established in both phases of the study. During the 20-year period the excess of male patients among oral cancer cases decreased significantly from 5.8:1 in the 1st phase to 3.7:1 in the 2nd phase.

Age distribution of the male and female patients was also examined in the two phases. During the examined period the mean age of female oral cancer cases increased from 62.2 years in the 1st phase to 63.5 years in the 2nd phase. The mean age of male oral cancer patients was significantly lower in the 1st phase (55.6 years) and showed further non-significant decrease in the second phase (54.1 years). These data justify an increasing difference of mean ages between male and female oral cancer cases. Young women (<40 yrs) among the oral cancer cases occurred rarely, they construed 4.5% of patients in the 1st phase and 3.9% in the 2nd phase. The ratio of similarly young male cases with oral cancer was significantly higher both in the 1st and 2nd phase and showed a slightly increasing trend (8.1% and 8.6%, respectively).

Intraoral location of cancers among men and women were separately evaluated in the two phases. In the 1st phase among male oral cancer cases the vermilion border and mucosa of the lower lip were the most common sites of involvement (35.0%). This was followed in decreasing order by the sublingual cancers (25.8%) tongue cancers (17.9%) and gingival cancers (11.3%). Other rare cancer locations (buccal mucosa, palate, upper lip, uvula) shared on the remaining 10%. In the 2nd phase among male oral cancer cases primacy of sublingual cancer (41.6%) was a conspicuous change. This was followed in decreasing order by the tongue cancers (24.6%) and the strongly decreased ratio of lower lip cancers (15.8%). The ratio of gingival cancers was relatively low (13.0%), showing however, a moderately increasing tendency (Figure 1.1).

In the 1st phase, among female oral cancer patients, gingival tumor location was the most frequent (23.9%). This was followed in order by lower lip cancer (18.5%), tongue cancer (18.3%) and sublingual cancer (14.1%). In the 2nd phase gingival cancers were in the leading position again, with their fairly increasing ratio (28.3%). They were closely followed by the sublingual (26.7%) and tongue cancers (23.9%). At the same time the ratio of lower lip cancer fairly diminished (8.9%) (Figure 1.2).

Smoking habits were registered in the groups of male and female patients with oral cancer and their controls in both phases. Patients were regarded as smokers if they actively used tobacco or had been smokers and abandoned it within 10 years.

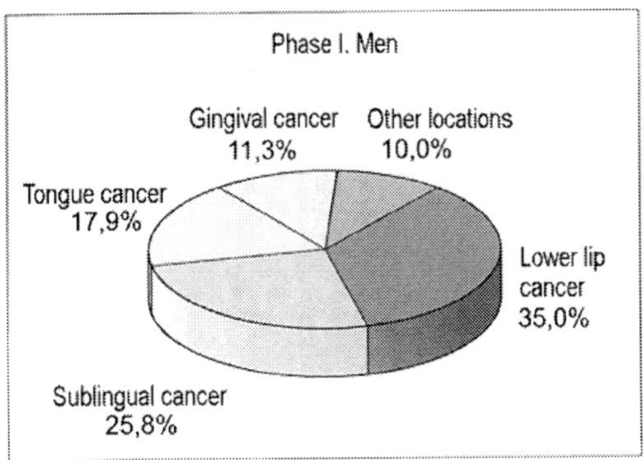

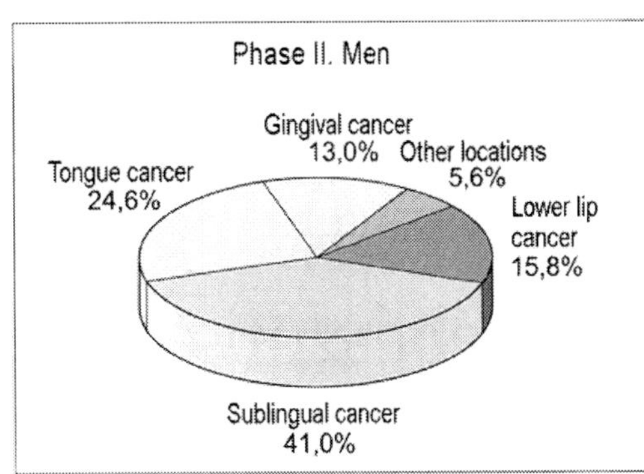

Figure 1.1. Distribution of oral cancer location among men in the two phases of the study.

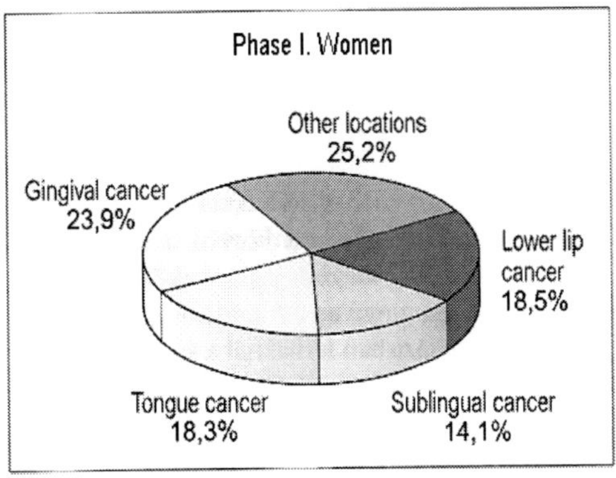

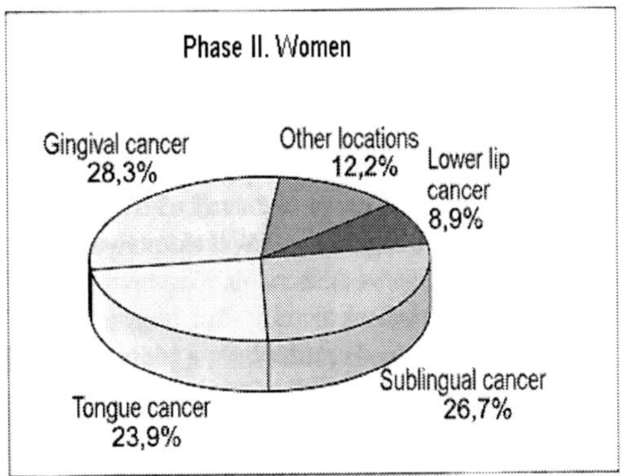

Figure 1.2. Distribution of oral cancer location among women in the two phases of the study.

In the group of tumor-free male control cases the ratio of smokers decreased from 57.5% in the 1st phase to 50.7% in the 2nd phase. Among the male cases with oral cancer the ratio of smokers was significantly higher as compared with their controls, though showed a decreasing tendency: 77.5% in the 1st phase and 73.5% in the 2nd phase.

Among the female tumor-free control cases the ratio of smokers also showed a decreasing tendency during the 20 years; being 44.4% in the 1st phase and 36.3% in the 2nd phase. Similarly, in the groups of women with oral cancer the ratio of smokers diminished from 58.2% in the 1st phase to 52.1% in the 2nd phase.

Alcohol consumption habits were evaluated in the groups of male and female patients in both phases. Abstinent cases and regular drinkers were discerned both among the oral cancer and control cases. Patients who confessed occasional alcohol consumption were regarded as non-drinkers.

Among the male tumor-free control cases the ratio of regular drinkers significantly decreased during the examination period; from 36.6% to 16.3%. Among the male patients with oral cancer the ratio of regular drinking was significantly higher as compared with their controls. However, during the 20 years a significant decrease in the ratio of regular drinkers could be observed among male cases with oral cancer; from 61.7% to 46.7%.

Among the female tumor-free controls the ratio of alcohol consumers was similarly low in both phases (4.0% and 3.9%, respectively). In the female oral cancer groups the alcohol consumption ratio was significantly higher as compared with the controls both in the first and second phase of the study; 10.5% and 11.5%. However, there was no significant change in the ratio of regular drinkers regarding either the oral cancer cases or controls during the twenty years.

Evaluation of the Epidemiological Changes in Oral Cancer Incidence in Hungary

The conspicuously high *male to female ratio* of the Hungarian oral cancer cases significantly decreased over the 20-year period. This decline of male to female ratio over decades is a global trend in the epidemiology of oral cancer; however, there are no rational explanations for this trend till now [11].

The *mean age* of female oral cancer patients was significantly higher as compared with males and this age difference became slightly more marked after a 20-year period. This gender related age difference of oral cancer cases has been a classical observation in many studies for a long time, but its reason could not be revealed so far [40,69].

Arteriosclerosis has well known associations with sexual steroids as the reproductive life of women seems to be protective, whereas postmenopausal loss of hormones is a risk for vascular diseases (see Chapter 4). Gender and age predilection of oral cancer cases is similar to that of cardiovascular diseases and these similarities suggest some hormonal influences on the development of this tumor. Among middle-aged cases with oral cancer a significantly higher prevalence of male patients as compared with females can be observed. However, after the mean age of female menopause (50 yrs) the risk for oral cancer slowly increases among women (see Chapter 5).

Researchers in Italy established that a low risk diet for cardiovascular diseases containing high rates of fish, vegetables and fruits shares in several aspects with a favorable diet against cancer [42]. This protective effect of the so-called Mediterranean diet was observed both against cancers of the upper digestive tract and other non-digestive epithelial neoplasms. Supposedly, these advantageous effects of a healthy diet may be explained not only by the intraoral local effects but also by the systemic increase in insulin sensitivity and in antioxidant capacity (see Chapter 2).

Postmenopausal women have strong progressive inclination to disorders of the glucose metabolism, which are common risk factors both for cardiovascular diseases and malignancies [89]. Recently, these hormonal and metabolic changes proved to be risk factors for oral cancer among Hungarian patients [78].

The distribution of *intraoral cancer sites* and its temporary changes may supply valuable data concerning the etiological factors of oral tumors.

Trends of changes in tumor site predilection among oral cancer cases showed a significantly decreasing prevalence of *lower lip cancer* both in the male and female patient groups. This is a well-known global trend and may be associated with the decrease of outdoor occupations. Windy weather and the ultraviolet spectrum of excessive sunshine may cause dryness and atrophy of the vermilion (chronic solar cheilitis), which is regarded as a precancerous state.

A further important finding is the progressive increase of *sublingual cancer* incidence both in male and female groups of oral cancer cases, which is also a global trend. This intraoral tumor location has the closest association with exogenous carcinogenic noxae. These harmful compounds may be others than tobacco and alcohol derivatives, such as environmental pollution, food additives, pesticides and so on. Carcinogenic compounds are concentrated in the saliva and along the salivary flow in the sublingual region and on the ventral surface of the tongue they may exert a contact toxic effect [61].

Separate analysis of the frequency of tumor sites in the male and female groups revealed gender related differences. Among the male oral cancer patients the lower lip location had a primacy in the first phase of the study, overtaken in the second phase by sublingual cancer. Among female oral cancer cases gingival cancer was a consequently leading site in both phases of the study.

Gingival cancer prevalence exhibited the most conspicuous difference between the male and female patient groups. It was the most frequent tumor location in women both in the first and second phase of the investigation and showed an increasing trend. On the contrary, in the male oral cancer groups of the two phases the gingival cancer ratio was conspicuously lower than the female cases and showed a moderate increase.

Gingival and periodontal tissues are fairly hormone sensitive [56]. Both postmenopausal state and type-2 diabetes are frequently associated with gingivitis and periodontitis. The gender related differences in gingival cancer incidence suggest that in older women these chronic inflammatory processes may have a role in cancer development.

In the two phases of our study, comparison of the smoking habits of the oral cancer cases and the tumor free controls may supply important information. The aim was to explore whether the permanently increasing morbidity and mortality of oral cancer in Hungary may be closely associated with the smoking habits of the general population or involvement of other factors might be assumed.

The present results established that the *ratio of smokers* showed a decreasing tendency during the studied 20 years both among the oral cancer cases and their tumor-free controls. However, the ratio of smokers in the oral cancer groups of both the male and female cases was significantly higher as compared with the control patients.

A markedly decreasing trend of *alcohol consumer ratio* was observed during the 20 years both in the tumor-free control and oral cancer groups of male cases. However, the ratio of regular alcohol consumers in the oral cancer groups of male cases was significantly higher as compared with the controls in both phases. These results suggest that alcohol consumption remained a risk factor for oral cancer among the male cases; however, the increasing trend of oral cancer incidence in Hungary has no associations with changes in the rate of alcohol abusers.

Among the female tumor-free control cases the rather low ratio of regular alcohol consumers did not show marked changes during the 20 years. In the group of women with oral cancer a significantly higher rate of drinkers was found as compared with their tumor-free controls. However, comparison of rates of alcohol consumers in the female oral cancer groups of the two phases did not show marked change after 20 years.

These data suggest that the extraordinarily rapid increase in oral cancer morbidity and mortality in Hungary is not reasonable simply on the basis of the Hungarian tobacco and alcohol consumption habits.

The Hungarian population is afflicted by multiple disadvantageous factors, which mean high risks for the development of cancers. The unfavorable socioeconomic circumstances after the 2nd World War became more severe following the thorough political and economical changes in 1989.

Economical troubles may result in increased cancer risk by several pathways. The continental position of Hungary and the long winters result in the extreme expensiveness of fruits and vegetables. Cheap, unhealthy diets rich in carbohydrates and saturated fats are high risk factors for oral cancer. Moreover, the insurance-based dental care was cancelled in the early 90s in Hungary and lack of regular dentistry check-ups and neglected teeth are all proven risk factors for oral malignancies.

Low income, large-scale impoverishment, fear of unemployment and homelessness became everyday reasons for anxiety and stress for the majority of Hungarian people, which all have indirect effect on cancer development as well. Considering all these factors they fairly contribute to the increased morbidity and mortality of oral cancer in Hungary in spite of the decreasing trend of smoking and drinking.

Changes in the male to female ratio of oral cancer after 20 years, the consequently older age of female patients as compared with males and the gender related difference of the prevalent tumor sites suggest some role of gender specific, systemic risk factors for oral cancer.

Necessity to Search for Further Cancer Risk Factors

Oral cancer is a multicausal disease and there are thorough interrelationships among the etiologic factors. Till now the exogenous harmful noxae (tobacco, alcohol consumption and energy rich diet) were overemphasized in oral cancer epidemiology [3,37,43,61,69].

Nevertheless, exogenous dietary factors, tobacco and alcohol consumption have not only local carcinogenic effect in the oral cavity, but also induce systemic changes by means of metabolic and hormonal pathways (see Chapters 2 and 8). Inflammation, atrophy and hyperplastic processes on the epithelial surface of the oral mucosa caused by external, internal factors or both, may enhance the vulnerability of the squamous epithelial cells and may provoke disturbances in their regeneration [56].

With full knowledge of these correlations, isolated investigations of exogenous risk factors may be misleading, without yielding correct results. The controversial associations and trends in oral cancer epidemiology focused the attention to search for further possible risk factors.

Recently, our working group established in case control studies that insulin resistance, such as metabolic syndrome, type-2 diabetes and estrogen deficiency seem also to be high risk factors for oral tumors [77,79,84]. These newly recognized cancer risk factors and their correlations with further regulatory mechanisms will be discussed in the following chapters.

References

[1] Atula S, Grénman R, Laippala P, Syrjänen S: Cancer of the tongue in patients younger than 40 years. *Arch Otolaryngol. Head Neck Surg.* 122:1313-1319, 1996

[2] Bagnardi V, Blangiardo M, LaVecchia C, Corrao G: A meta-analysis of alcohol drinking and cancer risk. *Br. J. Cancer*, 85:1700-1705, 2001

[3] Binnie WH, Rankin KV, Mackenzie IC: Etiology of oral squamous cell carcinoma. *J. Oral Path* 12:11-29, 1983

[4] Balaram P, Sridhar H, Rajkumar T, Vaccarella S, Herrero R, Nandakumar A, Ravichandran K, Ramdas K, Sankaranarayanan R, Gajalakshmi V, Munoz N, Franceschi S: Oral cancer in southern India: the influence of smoking, drinking, paan-chewing and oral hygiene. *Int. J. Cancer* 98:440-445, 2002

[5] Blask DE, Brainard GC, Dauchy RT, Hanifin JP, Davidson LK, Krause JA, Sauer LA, Rivera-Bermudez MA, Dubocovich ML, Jasser SA, Lynch DT, Rollag MD, Zalatan F: Melatonin-depleted blood from premenopausal women exposed to light at night stimulates growth of human breast cancer xenografts in nude rats. *Cancer Res.* 65:11174-11184, 2005

[6] Bosetti C, Franceschi S, Negri E, Talamini R, Tomei F, LaVecchia C: Changing socioeconomic correlates for cancers of the upper digestive tract. *Annals Oncol.* 12:327-330, 2001.

[7] Byers RM: Squomous Cell Carcinoma of the oral tongue in patients less than thirty years of age. *The American Journal of Surgery* 130:475-478, 1975

[8] Carniol PJ, Fried MP: Head and neck carcinoma in patients under 40 years of age. *Ann. Otolaryngol.* 91:152-155, 1982

[9] Chang MC, Chang CP, Lee JJ, Hahn LJ, Jeng JH: Cell-mediated immunity and head and neck cancer; with special emphasis on betel quid chewing habit. *Oral Oncol.* 41:757-775, 2005

[10] Chen J, Eisenberg E, Krutchkoff DJ, Katz RV: Changing trends in oral cancer in the United States, 1935 to 1985: A Connecticut Study. *J. Oral Maxillofac Surg.* 49:1152-1158, 1991

[11] Clayman, L: Oral cancer. A practical guide to understanding oral cancer. ELLM Press, 2002

[12] Cusumano RJ, Persky MS: Squamous cell carcinoma of the oral cavity and oropharynx in young adults. *Head Neck Surg.* 10:229-234, 1988

[13] da Silva CE, da Silva ID, Cerri A, Weckx LL: Prevalence of human papillomavirus in squamous cell carcinoma of the tongue. *Oral Surg. Oral Med. Oral Pathol. Oral Rad. Endodont*, 104:497-500, 2007

[14] Davis S, Severson RK: Increasing incidence of cancer of the tongue in the United States among young adults. *The Lancet* 2:910-911, 1987

[15] Decker J, Goldstein JC: Risk factors in head and neck cancer. *N Engl. J. Med.* 306:1151-1155, 1982

[16] Döbrőssy L. Cancer mortality in central-eastern Europe: Facts behind the figures. *Lancet Oncol.* 3:374-381, 2002

[17] Döbrössy L: Epidemiology of oral tumors. Fogorv Szle (in Hungarian) 100:47-52, 2007

[18] El-Naggar AK, Hurr K, Huff V, Luna MA, Goepfert H, Batsakis, JG: Allelic loss and replication errors at microsatellite loci on chromosome 11p in head and neck squamous carcinoma: association with aggressive biological features. *Clin. Cancer Res.* 2:903-907, 1996

[19] Fleming D, Shear M, Altini M: Intraoral squamous cell carcinoma in South Africa. J. *Dental Assoc. South Africa* 37:541-544, 1982

[20] Franceschi S, Talamini R, Barra S, Baron AE, Negri E, Bidoli E et al: Smoking and drinking in relation to cancers of the oral cavity, pharynx, larynx and esophagus in Northern Italy. *Cancer Res.* 50:6502-6507, 1990

[21] Franceschi S, Bidoli E, Baron AE, Talamini R, Serraino D, La Vecchia C: Nutrition and cancer of the oral cavity and pharynx in north-east Italy. *Int. J. Cancer* 47:20-25, 1991

[22] Franco EL, Kowalski LP, Oliveira BV, Curado MP, Pereira RN, Silva ME et al: Risk factors for oral cancer in Brazil. A case-control study. *Int. J. Cancer* 43:992-1000, 1989

[23] Garrote LF, Herrero R, Reyes RM, Vaccarella S, Anta JL, Ferbeye L, Munoz N. Franceschi S: Risk factors for cancer of the oral cavity and oro-pharynx in Cuba. *Br. J. Cancer* 85: 46-54, 2001.

[24] Gaudi I, Kásler M: Changes in mortality from malignant tumors between 1975 and 2001. Magyar Onkológia (English abstr) 46:291-295, 2002

[25] Gillison ML, Shah KV: Human papillomavirus-associated head and neck squamous cell carcinoma: mounting evidence for an etiologic role for human papillomavirus in a subset of head neck cancers. *Curr. Opin. Oncol.* 13:183-188, 2001

[26] Gillison ML: Current topics in the epidemiology of oral cavity and oropharyngeal cancers. *Head and Neck* 29:779-792, 2007

[27] Gridley G, McLaughlin JK, Block G, Blot WJ, Gluch M, Fraumeni F JrJ: Vitamin supplement use and reduced risk of oral and pharyngeal cancer. *Am. J. Epidemiol.* 135:1083-1092, 1992

[28] Gupta PC: Mouth cancer in India: a new epidemic? *J. Indian Med. Assoc.* 97:370, 1999

[29] Hofmann N, Tillonen J, Rintamaki H, Salapuro M, Lindquist C, Meurman JH: Poor dental status increases acetaldehyde-production from ethanol in saliva: a possible link to increased oral cancer risk in heavy drinkers. *Oral Oncol*, 37:153-158, 2001

[30] Iype EM, Pandey M, Mathew A, Thomas G, Sebastian P, Nair MK: Oral cancer among patients under the age of 35 years. *J. Postgrad Med.* 47:171-176, 2001

[31] Johnson NW, Warnakulasuriya KAAS: Epidemiology and aetiology of oral cancer in the United Kingdom. *Commun. Dental Health* 10:13-29, 1993

[32] Johnson NW: Etiology and risk factors for oral cancer, with special reference to- bacco and alcohol use. *Hungarian Oncol.* (English abstr) 45:115-122, 2001

[33] Johnson N: Tobacco use and oral cancer: a global perspective. *J. Dent. Educ.* 65:328-339, 2001

[34] Jones JB, Lampe HB, Cheung HW: Carcinoma of the tongue in young patients. *The J. Otolaryngol.* 18:105-108, 1989

[35] Jovanovic A, Sculten EA, Kostense PJ, Snow GB, van der Waal I: Tobacco and alcohol related to the anatomical site of oral squamous cell carcinoma. *J. Oral Pathol. Med.* 22:459-462, 1993

[36] Józan P: Health crisis east of the Elbe: a consequence of modernization? ACP News 1996

[37] Kademani D: Oral cancer. *Mayo Clin. Proc.* 82:878-887, 2007

[38] Koch WM, Lango M, Sewell D et al: Head and neck cancer in nonsmokers: a distinct clinical and molecular entity. *Laryngoscope* 109:1544-1551, 1999

[39] Kogevinas M, Pearce N, Susser M, Boffetta P: Social inequalities and cancer. Lyon: IARC Press, 1997

[40] Krolls SO, Hoffman S: Squamous cell carcinoma of the oral soft tissues: a statistical analysis of 14,253 cases by age, sex, and race of patients. *JADA* 92:571-574, 1976

[41] Kuriakose M, Sankaranarayanan M, Nair MK, Cherian T, Sugar AW, Scully C et al: Comparison of oral squamous cell carcinoma in younger and older patients in India. *Oral Oncology European Journal Cancer* 28B:113-120, 1992

[42] La Vecchia C, Chatenoud L, Altieri A, Tavani A: Nutrition and health: epidemiology of diet, cancer and cardiovascular disease in Italy. *Nutr. Met. and Cariovasc. Dis.* 11:10-15, 2001

[43] La Vecchia C, Lucchini F, Negri E, Levi F: Trends in oral cancer mortality in Europe. *Oral Oncol.* 40:433-439, 2004

[44] La Vecchia C: Mediterranean diet and cancer. (Review). *Public Health Nutr.* 7:965-968, 2004

[45] Levi F, Lucchini F, Negri E, Zatonski W, Boyle P, La Vecchia C: Trends in cancer mortality in the European Union and accession countries, 1980-2000. *Ann. Oncol.* 15: 1425-1431, 2004

[46] Lewin F, Norell SE, Johansson H et al: Smoking tobacco, oral snuff, and alcohol in the etiology of squamous cell carcinoma of the head and neck: a population-based case-referent study in Sweden. *Cancer* 82:1367-1375, 1998

[47] Lipkin A, Miller RH, Woodson GE: Squamous cell carcinoma of the oral cavity, pharynx and larynx in young adults. *Laryngoscope* 95:790-793, 1985

[48] Lissowska J, Pilarska A, Pilarski P, Samolczyk-Wanyura D, Piekarczyk J, Bardin-Mikollajczak A, Zatonski W, Herrero R, Munoz N, Franceschi S: Smoking, alcohol, diet, dentition and sexual practices in the epidemiology of oral cancer in Poland. *Eur. J. Cancer Prev.* 12:25-33, 2003

[49] Llewellyn CD, Johnson NW, Warnakulasuriya KAAS: Risk factors for squamous cell carcinoma of the oral cavity in young people-a comprehensive literature review. *Oral Oncol.* 37:401-418, 2001

[50] Llewellyn CD, Linklater K, Bell J, Johnson NW, Warnakulasuriya KA: Squamous cell carcinoma of the oral cavity in patients aged 45 years and under: a descriptive analysis of 116 cases diagnosed in the South East of England from 1990 to 1997. *Oral Oncol.* 39:106-114, 2003

[51] Llewellyn CD, Johnson NW, Warnakulasuriya KA: Risk factors for oral cancer in newly diagnosed patients aged 45 years and younger: a case-control study in Southern England. *J. Oral Pathol. Med.* 33:525-532, 2004

[52] Lydiatt WM, Davidson BJ, Shah J, Schantz SP, Chaganti RSK: The relationship of loss of heterozygosity to tobacco exposure and early recurrence in head and neck squamous cell carcinoma. *J. Surg.* 168:437-440, 1994

[53] Macfarlane GJ, Boyle P: Rising mortality from cancer of the tongue in young Scottish males. *The Lancet* 2:912,Abstract 1987

[54] Marshall J, Graham S, Mettlin C, Shedd D, Swanson M: Diet in the epidemiology of oral cancer. *Nutrition and Cancer* 3:145-149, 1982

[55] McGregor GI, Davis N, Robbins RE: Squamous cell carcinoma of the tongue and lower oral cavity in patients under 40 years of age. *Am. J. Surg.* 146:88-92, 1983

[56] Mealey BL, Moritz AJ: Hormonal influences: effects of diabetes mellitus and endogenous female sex steroid hormones on the periodontium. *Periodontology* 2000. 32:59-81, 2003

[57] Merrill RM, Isakson RT, Beck RE: The association between allergies and cancer: what is currently know? *Ann. Allergy Asthma Immunol.* 99:102-116; quiz 117-119, 150, 2007

[58] Mork J, Lie AK, Glattre E et al: Human papillomavirus infection as a risk factor for squamous-cell carcinoma of the head and neck. *N Engl. J. Med.* 344:1125-1131, 2001

[59] Myers JN, Elkins T, Roberts D, Byers RM: Squamous cell carcinoma of tongue in young adults: increasing incidence and factors that predict treatment outcomes. *Otolaryngol. Head Neck Surg.* 122:44-51, 2000

[60] Narito T, Kudo H: Effect of melatonin on B16 melanoma growth in athymic mice. *Cancer Res.* 45:4175-4177, 1985

[61] Neville BW, Day TA: Tumors and precancerous lesions of the oral cavity. CA *Cancer J. Clin.* 52:195-215, 2002

[62] Newman AN, Rice DH Ossoff RH, Sisson GA: Carcinoma of tongue in persons younger than 30 years of age. *Arch Otolaryngol.* 109:302-304, 1983

[63] Okamoto Y, Hayashi T, Toda C, Ueda K, Hashizume K, Itoh K, Nishikawa J, Nishihara T, Kojima N: Formation of estrogenic products from environmental phthalate esters under light exposure. *Chemosphere*, 64: 1785-1792, 2006

[64] Otto Sz: Cancer epidemiology in Hungary and the Béla Johan National Program for the Decade of Health. *Path Oncol. Res.* 9: 126-130, 2003

[65] Padmanabham TK, Sankaranarayanan M, Nair MK: Evaluation of local control, survival and pattern of failure with radiotherapy in cancer of the tongue. *Oncology* 47:121-123, 1990

[66] Parkin DM, Pisani P, Ferlay J: Estimates of the worldwide incidence of eighteen major cancers in 1985. *Int. J. Cancer* 54:594-606, 1993

[67] Poschl G, Seitz HK: Alcohol and Cancer. *Alcohol and Alcoholism* 39:155-165, 2004

[68] Reibel J: Tobacco and oral diseases: update on the evidence, with recommendations. *Med. Princ. Pract.* 12:22-32, 2003

[69] Rich AM, Radden BG: Squamous cell carcinoma of the oral mucosa: a review of 244 cases in Australia. *J. Oral. Pathol.* 13:459-471, 1984

[70] Rohr UD, Herold J: Melatonin deficiencies in women. Maturitas, 41 Suppl 1, S85-S104, 2002

[71] Rosenquist K, Wennerberg J, Schildt EB, Bladstrom A, Goran HB, Andersson G: Oral status, oral infections and some lifestyle factors as risk factors for oral and oropharyngeal squamous cell carcinoma. A population-based case-control study in southern Sweden. *Acta Otolaryngol.* 125:1327-1336, 2005

[72] Rossing MA, Vaughan TL, McKnight B: Diet and pharyngeal cancer. *Int. J. Cancer* 44:593-597, 1989

[73] Sankaranarayanan R, Mohideen MN, Nair MK, Padmanabhan TK: Aetiology of oral cancer in patients <30 years of age. *Brit. J. Cancer* 59:439-440, 1989

[74] Schantz SP, Yu GP: Head and neck cancer incidence trends in young Americans, 1973-1997, with a special analysis for tongue cancer. *Arch Otolaryngol. Head Neck Surg.* 128:268-274, 2002

[75] Singh B, Bhaya M, Zimbler M et al: Impact of comorbidity on outcome of young patients with head and neck squamous cell carcinoma. *Head Neck* 20:1-7, 1998

[76] Streilein JW: Immunogenetic factors in skin cancer. *New Engl. J. Med.* 325:884-887, 1991

[77] Suba Zs, Barabás J, Szabó Gy, Takács D, Ujpál M: Increased prevalence of diabetes and obesity in patients with salivary gland tumors. *Diabetes Care* 28:228, 2005

[78] Suba Zs, Barabás J: Prevention of oral cancer (in hungarian) pp. *Medicina* ZRT, Budapest, 2007

[79] Suba Zs: Gender-related hormonal risk factors for oral cancer. *Pathol Oncol. Res.* 13: 195-202, 2007

[80] Subapriya R, Thangavelu A, Mathavan B, Ramachandran CR, Nagini S: Assessment of risk factors for oral squamous cell carcinoma in Chidambaram, Southern India: a case-control study. *Eur. J. Cancer Prev.* 16:251-256, 2007

[81] Szabó Gy, Klenk G, Veér A: Correlation of the combination of alcoholism and smoking with the occurrence of cancer in the oral cavity. A screnning study in the endangered population. Mund Kiefer Gesichtschir (in German) 3:119-121, 1999

[82] Tezal M, Sullivan MA, Reid ME, Marshall JR, Hyland A, Loree T, Lillis C, Hauck L, Wactawski-Wende J, Scannapieco FA: Chronic periodontitis and the risk of tongue cancer. *Head Neck Surg.* 133:450-454, 2007

[83] Tsukuda M, Ooishi K, Mochimatsu I, Sato H: Head and neck carcinomas in patients under the age of forty years. *Japanese J. of Cancer Res.* 84:748-752, 1993

[84] Ujpál M, Matos O. Bíbok Gy, Somogyi A, Szabó Gy, Suba Zs: Diabetes and oral tumors in Hungary: Epidemiological correlations. Diabetes Care 27:770-774, 2004.

[85] Varga E, Tyldsley WR: Carcinoma arising in cyclosporin-induced gingival hyperplasia. *Brit. Dental J.* 171:26.27, 1991

[86] Wang Y, Spitz MR, Lee JJ, Huang M, Lippman SM, Wu X: Nucleotide excision repair pathway genes and oral premalignant lesions. *Clin. Cancer Res*, 13:3753-3758, 2007

[87] Warnakulasuriya KAAS: Cancers of the oral cavity and pharynx. In: Vogelstein B, Kinzler Keds. The genetic basis of human cancer. McGrow Hill, New York, 2001.

[88] Winn DM, Zeigler RG, Pickle LW, Gridley G, Blot WJ, Hoover RN: Diet in the etiology of oral and pharyngeal cancer among women from the Southern United States. *Cancer Res.* 44:1216-????

[89] Wu ShI, Chou P, Tsai ShT: The impact of years since menopause on the development of impaired glucose tolerance. *J. Clin. Epidemiol.* 54:117-120, 2001

[90] Wynder EL, Bross IJ, Feldman RM: A study of the etiological factors in cancer of the mouth. Cancer 10:1300-1323, 1957

[91] Zheng W, Blot WJ, Diamond EL, Norkus EP, Spate V, Morris JS et al: Serum micronutrients subsequent risk of oral and pharyngeal cancer. *Cancer Res.* 53:795-798, 1993.

Chapter 2

Insulin Resistance, Hyperinsulinemia and Cancer Risk

How innocent is a Bystander? (Zimmet)

Insulin resistance is a defect of the insulin-mediated cellular glucose uptake, which may elicit many disorders in gene regulation of cell metabolism, growth, differentiation and mitotic activity [16,60].

The discovery of insulin resistance as a complex metabolic disturbance was a milestone in understanding human illnesses [103]. Insulin resistance is a worldwide risk factor for the two most dangerous disease groups; namely for cardiovascular lesions and malignancies [15,16].

In the first, compensated phase of insulin resistance the serum glucose level is maintained within the normal range at the expense of a reactive hyperinsulinemia. Elevated insulin level in itself is an increased cancer risk [52] and it may enhance the production and mitogenic activity of other, insulin-like growth factors, such as IGF-I and IGF-II, which have important role in cell proliferation and tumor induction at several sites [136]. In the second, uncompensated phase of insulin resistance the secretor capacity of insular β-cells is exhausted and with increasing plasma glucose level, metabolic syndrome and type-2 diabetes develop. Elevated fasting glucose level has also tumor provoking effects by several pathways [89].

All phases of insulin resistance (hyperinsulinemia, hyperglycemia, metabolic syndrome and type-2 diabetes) are proven risk factors for pancreas, liver, colon, kidney urinary bladder, prostate, salivary gland and oral cavity cancers and even for malignancies of the highly estrogen dependent tissues (breast, ovary, endometrium) [1,7,27,63,77,84,89,118,120,129, 135]. These associations are to be systematically explored for further cancer types.

Correlation of Metabolic Syndrome (Insulin Resistance Syndrome) with Cancer Risk

A famous hypothesis of Reaven notified in 1988 established a causal association between insulin resistance and hyperinsulinaemia, which are basic disorders for many human diseases [103]. Earlier, cardiovascular illnesses were regarded as complications of type-2 diabetes. However, the new theory revealed that many divergent symptoms and findings, such as hypertension, dyslipidemia, elevated fasting glucose and hyperuricemia all have a common soil; the insulin resistance [28]. This new clinical entity was named as metabolic X syndrome [104], obesity was later associated to the basic features. The metabolic syndrome is a complex systemic disorder with continuous progression and proved to be a high risk factor for type-2 diabetes, cardiovascular diseases and malignancies [15].

Insulin is produced by the β-cells of pancreatic islands and transported by the blood stream and may exert its activities in remote tissues. Insulin receptors are expressed on all cell types, even on tumor cells. The most important function of insulin is the facilitation of the anabolic processes [61]. It activates many transport systems being associated with the metabolism of carbohydrates, lipids and proteins, and at the same time hampers the catabolic processes, which are regulated by antagonistic hormone systems.

Insulin resistance results in divergent pathologic processes, which produce disturbances not only in the cellular glucose uptake but also in the lipid and protein metabolism, in hemostasis and in cation-transport. As insulin is at the same time a growth factor, alterations of the late postreceptor processes in insulin resistance may disturb both cell growth and cell proliferation [62].

Nowadays, metabolic syndrome has great impact as it shows an epidemic spread in the developed countries. "Western lifestyle" (obesity, lack of physical activity and carbohydrate-lipid rich diet) favors for the development of insulin resistance and for its severe consequences [42]. There is a worldwide reasonable effort to reveal the mechanisms, which lead to insulin resistance and to find the possibilities for preventive measures.

Today, basic criteria of the metabolic syndrome are hyperglycemia, visceral obesity, hypertension, elevated triglyceride level, and low HDL-cholesterol level [105]. Each component of the metabolic syndrome has individually been linked in some way to the development of cancer. Together, they may all represent a multiple cancer risk beyond that of the individual components alone [27]. Nowadays, we are on the way to regard malignancies as complications of insulin resistance. The metabolic syndrome is a high-risk state not only for cardiovascular diseases but also for cancers.

Hyperinsulinemia and Cancer Risk

In the first, partially compensated phase of insulin resistance increased activity of the β-cells of pancreas islands endeavours to maintain the physiologic serum glucose level at the expense of hyperinsulinemia. However, this compensatory mechanism has a great risk [62].

Some mutations of insulin receptors result in loss of the stimulative effect on glucose transport and glycogen synthesis, however the mitogenic and antiapoptotic effect is preserved

[61]. This reveals that insulin mediated cellular processes are fairly divergent and do not have parallel vulnerability [65]. When insulin resistance affects the insulin mediated glucose uptake selectively and the growth factor activity remains unaltered, a reactive hyperinsulinemia may provoke pathologic cell proliferation [94].

There are contradictory data on the tumor provoking effect of hyperinsulinemia, as insulin besides metabolic and growth factor activities may increase the production and mitogenic activity of other insulin-like growth factors (IGFs) and epidermal growth factor [65,92,95]. As insulin shares in the activation of cell proliferation with IGFs, one can hardly establish whether it is a sinner, an assassin or an innocent bystander on the pathway of the pathologic processes [137].

Mediators leading to malignant transformation may include activation of tyrosine kinase and mitogen-activated protein kinase (MAPK) pathways by insulin binding to its receptor [30]. As insulin stimulates the cell cycle, overexpression of insulin receptors and malignant transformation may be closely associated. Besides enhanced mitotic activity, increased DNA-synthesis, antiapoptotic effect and disturbance of the sexual steroid equilibrium may also contribute to the insulin mediated tumor-provoking effect. Close mutual associations of insulin effects and sexual steroids are discussed in Chapter 7.

Literary data support that obesity and type-2 diabetes associated with hyperinsulinemia are high risks for incidence of breast and colorectal cancers [29,57,66].

An elevated insulin level increases local tumor invasion, metastatic spread and mortality. Literary data justify the fatal progression of glandular epithelial cancers, such as liver, pancreas and prostate tumors caused by high serum insulin level, however, similar correlations were not found in pharyngeal and laryngeal tumor cases [7]. The prognosis of malignant tumors in patients with type-2 diabetes is generally worse as compared with non-diabetic cases, though the insulin levels might be fairly different. In type-2 diabetes cases colon and breast cancers emerged 8-10 years after diagnosis of the metabolic disorder. This finding suggests that earlier, long lasting hyperinsulinaemia may result in malignant processes [84,89]. Prognostic expectations of patients with prostate cancer and associated hyperinsulinemia proved to be unfavourable; the ratio of both metastatic spread and mortality were significantly high as compared with non-diabetic cancer cases [53].

There are several methods to decrease the serum insulin level. Enhanced physical activity, weight loss and Mediterranean diet lower both insulin level and cancer risk [85,90]. Insulin sensitivity may be increased by drug administration as well, resulting in lower insulin level. These methods are also promising in regard to tumor prevention and therapy.

Insulin-Like Growth Factors and Cancer Risk

Insulin resistance and hyperinsulinemia mean concomitantly elevated serum levels of IGFs. The crucial role of these growth factors is the regulation of pre- and postnatal development and the aging process. They regulate the growth, proliferation, differentiation and even malignant transformation of cells [23,92,132]. Epidemiological observations suggest that serum levels of IGFs and IGF-binding globulins are closely associated with cancer promotion [52,76,90,136]. The level of bioavailable IGF-1 without protein binding determines the carcinogenic capacity. High IGF-1 and low IGF-l-binding protein levels mean a high risk for breast, prostate and colon cancers [110].

The IGF-1 level in the circulation depends on the mutual interrelationship of genetic and environmental influences. The IGF-1 level is thoroughly modified by diet and lifestyle. Exclusively plant containing vega diet and a completely meat-free vegetarian diet markedly decrease the IGF-1 level in the circulation, which means a lower cancer risk [3]. An energy rich diet enhances the bioavailable IGF-1 level and at the same time increases the risk of cancers [50]. Excessive consumption of sweets with high glycemic index is also an increased cancer risk at several sites, supposedly by means of mobilization of insulin and IGF-1 together [5,6,124].

Lifestyle is also a determinant factor for IGF-1 level. Western lifestyle and lack of physical activity increase, whereas active sport decreases the concentration of bioavailable IGFs. Epidemiological studies revealed that physical activity decreases the risk for breast colon and prostate cancers and might even improve the prognosis of advanced tumors [85,90]. This effect can be attributed at least partially to the decreased level of circulatory IGFs.

The IGF system and insulin are in close interrelationship. The chemical structure of IGF-1 is similar to that of insulin and both have mitogenic and antiapoptotic effects [22]. IGF-1 can bind to the insulin receptor with a lower affinity and decreased effect. There are also hybrid receptors with binding capacity for both signals. Recently, new therapeutic possibilities emerged against malignant tumors by means of IGF-1-receptor blocking [112].

Hyperglycemia and Cancer Risk

Elevated fasting glucose level in the uncompensated stage of insulin resistance is a high risk for cancer by means of several pathways (see Chapter 3). Similarly, excessive intake of carbohydrates with high glycemic index may also promote carcinogenesis. Excessive glucose supply has direct influence on pathological cell proliferations and may indirectly provoke tumor initiation and growth by increased production of glucose transporters, reactive oxygen species, advanced glycation end products (AGEs), cytokines, IGFs and other mediators. Correlations between high fasting glucose level, type-2 diabetes and cancer risk are discussed in Chapter 3.

Visceral Obesity and Cancer Risk

Obesity is a well-known component of the metabolic syndrome and has close correlations with dyslipidemia hypertension and type-2 diabetes [81]. Central or visceral type obesity has close associations with metabolic alterations and is regarded as promoting factor for insulin resistance. Recently, obesity is regarded as high risk for both cardiovascular diseases and malignancies [59].

The mass of visceral fat tissue has decreased insulin sensitivity and the reactive hyperinsulinemia provokes excessive lipolysis [39]. The elevated free fatty acid (FFA) level primarily defines the correlations between obesity and insulin resistance. A great amount of FFA and lipoprotein may deliberate from the excessive visceral fatty tissue and enter into the portal circulation. High levels of FFA and lipoprotein do contribute to the development of dyslipidemia and result in glucose intolerance in the liver and peripheral muscles.

High lipid levels in the portal circulation decrease hepatic glucose uptake and storage and further increase insulin resistance [116]. Lower insulin sensitivity of the liver results in elevated glucose and insulin levels in the systemic circulation. These processes may be associated with the increased risk of type-2 diabetes and of atherogenic cardiovascular lesions. As the elevated serum levels of glucose, insulin and IGFs have crucial role in cancer promotion too, visceral obesity means a high tumor risk.

Correlations among visceral obesity, insulin resistance and tumor risk are strongly affected by the newly recognized endocrine function of the fatty tissue [83]. Excessive accumulation of the fatty tissue leads to an increased adipocytokine production (TNF-α, leptin, resistin, adiponectin, interleukin-6, etc.). These mediators thoroughly influence the insulin sensitivity and glucose metabolism as a base for the association between obesity and insulin resistance. Moreover, cytokines may maintain long lasting inflammatory processes. Some of them, e.g. TNF-α have a pivotal role in the promotion of insulin resistance in the peripheral tissues, and at the same time are players in the initiation and spread of some tumors [2,128].

Obesity also affects hormonal changes including estrogens, androgens, IGFs and insulin [24]. As obesity is in close correlation with insulin resistance, elevated insulin IFG and androgen levels are frequently observed both in male and female patients with high body mass index (BMI).

Recently, attention has been reasonably focused on estrogen as a potential mediator of obesity influenced cancer [63]. However, literary data on the associations between obesity induced cancer and estrogen level are fairly controversial. While postmenopausal obesity is strongly associated with increased breast cancer risk, particularly among women never using hormone replacement, obese premenopausal women may have decreased risk for breast cancer [16,89]. Moreover, a recent report found obesity to be most strongly related to mortality in women with estrogen receptor-negative breast cancers [36]. These data suggest that factors other than estrogen may mediate the correlations between obesity and breast cancer.

Obesity is often the predecessor of type-2 diabetes, cardiovascular diseases and several cancers. Weight loss may prevent the development of severe insulin resistance by favorable changes in lipid levels, decreased insulin, IGF and glucose levels and lower production of inflammatory cytokines. Caloric restriction decreases the incidence of breast cancer [87].

Epidemiological studies in Canada justified the causal role of obesity in 7.7% of all malignancies. Lymphoma, leukemia and cancers of the gastrointestinal tract, kidney, breast, pancreas, ovary and prostate were registered among the obesity-associated tumors [97].

Obesity thoroughly affects tumor progression as well. Obese patients are more likely to have lower physical activity and higher caloric and fat intakes when compared with non-obese cases. Advantageous effects of physical activity and weight loss were observed among obese patients with breast and colon cancers with decreased risk of local recurrences and metastatic spread of tumors and improved life expectancies [12,24,25].

Dyslipidemia and Cancer Risk

Insulin resistance and hyperinsulinemia are associated with a complex disturbance of the lipid metabolism and lead to dyslipidemia [104]. Nevertheless, fat administration in both in vivo and in vitro systems has been reported to induce insulin resistance [60].

Increased fatty acid levels stimulate fatty acid oxidation (both mitochondrial and peroxisomal), inhibit the cellular glucose uptake and promote gluconeogenesis. This may be the basis for fatty acid induced insulin resistance in the muscle and liver [60,97]. Dietary fat composition alters cell membrane phospholipid composition, insulin binding and glucose metabolism in the adipocytes of control and diabetic animals [41]. Moreover, dyslipidemia may interfere with changes in hormone signaling from the plasma membrane and cellular growth rate by alterations of the cell membrane composition [26].

Insulin resistance is associated with disturbances in lipolytic processes. This correlation results in a decreased lipoprotein lipase and increased hepatic lipase activity. In the metabolic syndrome, increased plasma level of very low-density lipoprotein (VLDL), low-density lipoprotein (LDL) and triglyceride, and decreased level of high-density lipoprotein (HDL) are characteristic findings [121]

The physiological insulin level hampers the deliberation of FFAs and decreases the fasting serum glucose level, which results in a favorable decrease in hepatic VLDL secretion. Insulin resistance is associated with elevated circulatory FFA and glucose levels, and VLDL production is also increased. A harmful decrease in HDL-cholesterol level is also associated with disturbance of the VLDL metabolism [116]

In the metabolic syndrome and in type-2 diabetes the triglyceride content of the lipoproteins is elevated. Serum level of triglycerides shows parallelism with insulin resistance, serum insulin level and BMI, whereas being inversely correlated with the HDL level. These data support that an elevated triglyceride level is the most reliable indicator of insulin resistance [104]. The causal factors of hypertriglyceridemia are the excessive substrate supply and the decreased activity of lipoprotein lipase. Lipid load in insulin resistant patients provokes high, long lasting hypertriglyceridemia and increased hepatic VLDL synthesis.

There are several pathways for correlations between lipid metabolism disorders and malignancies. Peroxisome proliferator activated receptors (PPARs) are regulated by lipid-associated signals, and they have pivotal roles in the development of insulin resistance, alterations of lipoprotein metabolism and their pathological consequences. Activated PPAR and a nuclear receptor retinoid-X (RXR) participate together in the regulation of transcription [80]. Increased activity of peroxisomes in lipid-oxidation processes may result in DNA-derangement leading to malignant transformation.

Lipid peroxidation may be involved in cancer development, and essential nutritients such as vitamins E and C have protective effect, as they are scavengers of free radicals. Significantly lower salivary levels of antioxidant vitamins were observed in oral cancer patients as compared with their controls [101]. Consequently, antioxidant nutrients may counteract free radical-mediated disturbances of cell proliferation.

Correlations of dyslipidemia and malignant tumors were thoroughly studied in colorectal and breast cancer cases [84,131]. Results of epidemiological and clinical examinations justified the close association between hypertriglyceridemia and tumor risk [84,89]. Excessive saturated fat ingestion, consecutive hypertriglyceridemia and insulin resistance proved to be risk factors for cancers at several sites.

Hypertension, Insulin Resistance and Cancer Risk

The pathophysiology of hypertension is not uniform; there may be many different mechanisms in the background. Hypertension usually shows close correlation with insulin resistance and hyperinsulinemia [51,71]. In patients with hypertension risk factors for cardiovascular diseases, such as insulin resistance, elevated insulin, fasting glucose, triglyceride and LDL levels, as well as low HDL level are characteristic findings [28]. There are crossroads between obesity and hypertension by means of hormonal regulation. A positive correlation between body mass index and angiotensinogen expression was reported in the subcutaneous adipose tissue of obese men [127].

Insulin has not only metabolic but also direct vasoactive effects, so the serum insulin level is in close positive correlation with the blood pressure [81,103]. In hyperinsulinemia vasopressor activities of insulin are more intensive than its vasodilatative impacts [34]. Insulin resistance and reactive hyperinsulinemia are closely associated with increased activity of the sympathetic nervous system, which results in vasoconstriction. Decreased blood flow in the skeletal muscles may further increase insulin resistance as a vicious circle. At the same time, decreased prostaglandin synthesis and nitrogen-oxide deliberation reduce vasodilatation. Insulin resistance increases the activity of the renin-angiotensin system and the more intense natrium reabsorption in the kidney tubules augment the plasma volume.

Excessive salt intake may negatively affect the insulin signal, which promotes insulin resistance [93] and also has great impact on the blood pressure. In the meantime, salt load also provokes cell growth by affecting the insulin signal system.

There are few literary data on the associations of hypertension and cancer promotion. However, results of some studies support that the prevalence of both cardiovascular diseases and malignant tumors is increased among patients with hypertension. Recently, epidemiological correlation between salivary gland tumors and hypertension was observed [119]. In postmenopausal women hypertension proved to be a strong risk factor for hormone-dependent tumors, separately from obesity [115]. Based on these data hypertension and cancer may be multifaceted tips on the deeply hidden iceberg of insulin resistance [28]

Dietary Habits, Insulin Resistance and Cancer Risk

Diet plays a definitive role in processes affecting the energy balance and metabolism. Dietary habits thoroughly influence not only oral health but also insulin sensitivity and cancer risk at several sites [72].

A low risk diet for cancer in the Mediterranean region implies increased consumption of fruit, vegetables and fish as well as avoiding excessive intakes of meat and refined carbohydrates [64,73]. Further, olive oil and other unsaturated fats are preferred to saturated ones. La Vecchia and coworkers studied the correlations between Mediterranean diet and cancers of the upper aerodigestive tract [18,45].

Mediterranean diet has benevolent anticancer effects not only on the gastrointestinal tract but also on other organs. Dietary protective effect of such a diet was also observed for breast, female genital tract, ovary, urinary tract and some other non-digestive epithelial neoplasms [17,72,73].

Healthy diet is associated with reduced IFG-I level and improvement of insulin sensitivity which also strengthens its anticancer capacity [130]. A favorable diet has an antioxidant potential and reduces the risk of both cardiovascular diseases and cancers of the oral, pharyngeal and laryngeal region [18,72].

Mediterranean diet may have favorable anticancer capacity even in strong smoker and drinker cases. Correlations of diet and risk of oral and pharyngeal cancer were studied in an Italian case-control study. The results provided further support to the beneficial effect of high intake of vegetables and fruits, particularly in heavy smokers and drinkers [123]. Data from a series of case-control studies conducted in 9 countries worldwide also revealed the advantageous modulation of the carcinogenic potential of tobacco and alcohol by the Mediterranean diet [67].

Many epidemiological data suggest that meals containing antioxidant vitamins (A, C, E) have benevolent systemic effects by decreasing the level of reactive free radicals [18]. Significantly lower levels of antioxidant vitamins E and C in the saliva were observed in oral cancer patients as compared with controls [101]. Recently, a direct link between salivary free radicals and oral squamous cell cancer has been demonstrated [10]. Age-related changes in salivary antioxidant profile and higher viscosity of the saliva in aged patients may also be associated with a higher oral cancer risk [55].

Whole grain food intake was consistently related to reduced cancer risk of several types of the upper digestive tract neoplasms. Epidemiological evidence of the relation between fiber-rich diet and colorectal cancer justified a protective effect [64,72,113]. In contrast, refined grain intake was associated with increased risk of cancers at different sites, suggesting a potential role of elevated IGF-1 level [72].

Recently, excessive consumption of sweet foods also emerged as a cancer risk factor. Load of foods with high glycemic index was found to be high risk for cancers of the oral cavity, stomach, breast, prostate and ovary [4,5,6,18,124]. The associations were similar for various cancer sites of the upper aerodigestive and colorectal tract [4,56]. The correlation between sweet food intake and cancer risk was stronger in women as compared with men, especially in those with high BMI. This latter observation suggests that obesity and the associated insulin resistance have closer correlation with glycemic load induced cancer in women as compared with men.

Dietary fat is an essential macronutritient, providing energy source and hydrophobic components for biomolecule synthesis. Fatty acids are also used for the synthesis of signaling molecules like steroid hormones [60]. Dietary fat has the potential to affect gene expression through multiple pathways leading to changes in carbohydrate and lipid metabolism as well as cancer initiation [109] Depending on the gene examined, polyunsaturated fatty acids (PUFAs) might augment or abrogate gene transcription, which leads to specific phenotypic changes altering cellular functions.

Low fat ingestion diets or diets that are disproportionately enriched in PUFAs have advantageous effect on gene expression leading to beneficial regulation of cellular metabolism, growth and differentiation [60]. Excessive saturated dietary fat intake may increase the levels of FFAs, triglycerides and low-density lipoprotein (LDL) cholesterol in the plasma. These changes provoke the onset and progression of insulin resistance and consequently elevate insulin and IGF levels. All these alterations are risk factors for both atherosclerotic diseases and malignancies [15,40,50,60,79,116].

Physical Activity, Insulin Resistance and Cancer Risk

Nowadays sport and physical activity are highly appreciated as important factors in both prevention and improvement of chronic diseases.

Diabetes mellitus has been regarded as a punishment of the civilized societies [20]. In the background of the metabolic syndrome and type-2 diabetes not only genetic determinants but also environmental factors have decisive role. Increased prevalence of obesity in the developed countries is regarded rather as a result of decreased physical activity than of excessive caloric intake.

Glucose uptake of the skeletal muscles depends on the glucose metabolism, the plasma glucose level and the membrane receptors of the sarcolemma. Physical activity and contraction of the muscle cells enhance the cellular glucose uptake even in case of a decreased insulin level [68]. Contraction of skeletal muscle fibers activates the GLUT-4 glucose transporter system. Glut-4 protein molecules are mobilized from the intracellular pools and show an increased expression on the membrane surfaces [107,111]. All these events support the close correlation between physical activity and insulin sensitivity.

In clinical studies, regular, moderate physical activity resulted in significantly increased glucose tolerance and decreased plasma insulin level in patients with type-2 diabetes [107]. Regular physical load results in loss of abdominal fat, decreased triglyceride and increased HDL level, as well as decrease of blood pressure [75]. Regular, daily walking may improve the insulin sensitivity, lipase activity, and fasting serum lipid and glucose levels. Changes in lifestyle were more effective on insulin sensitization as compared with metformin treatment [32].

As cancer prevalence is thoroughly associated with insulin resistance, physical activity has favorable impact both on prevention and treatment of malignancies [90]. Recreational physical activity decreased the breast cancer risk in postmenopausal women [25,86].

Darkness, Melatonin, Insulin Resistance and Cancer Risk

Darkness increases melatonin production, which is a pineal hormone. Controversial results concerning associations of melatonin and insulin resistance have been published [108]. In postmenopausal women application of melatonin reduced glucose tolerance and insulin sensitivity [21], which may be a route leading to increased tumor risk. Moreover, melatonin administration in perimenopausal women did produce changes in LH, FSH and thyroid hormone levels. In animal experiment some cancers started to grow after melatonin treatment [11]. Correlations of low exposure to light and increased cancer incidence in women may be at least partially mediated by reduced glucose tolerance.

Tobacco Use, Insulin Resistance and Cancer Risk

Smoking is a well-known etiological factor of both cardiovascular diseases and malignancies. Tobacco and its burn products are the most important exogenous carcinogenic factors and affect directly the upper aerodigestive tract such as the oral cavity, pharynx, larynx and bronchus [43,88].

Nicotine is a toxic component of cigarette smoke and inhibits nitrogen-oxide-induced apoptosis in the oral epithelial cells. Inhibition of NO-induced apoptosis may be an important participant of oral carcinogenesis [8]. Nicotine exposure might have a negative impact on the apoptotic potential of anticancer drugs resulting in a poor prognosis of oral cancer cases [134].

Smoking has not only local, carcinogenic capacities but also exerts thorough effect on metabolic processes and has strong correlations with cancers at sites other than the upper aerodigestive system. Moreover, it is the most important exogenous factor, which decreases the peripheral glucose uptake and provokes oxidative stress [37]. Nicotine and CO may provoke vasoconstriction and decrease deliberation of nitrogenoxyde as well as decreasing the peripheral blood flow in the skeletal muscles. These changes result in peripheral insulin resistance and hypertension.

In clinical studies current smokers exhibited an increased prevalence of metabolic syndrome and type-2 diabetes as compared with never smokers [35,49,58]. Smoking habits in middle-aged men strictly correlated with the degree of insulin resistance including increased levels of insulin, LDL-cholesterol, as well as triglycerides [35]. Insulin resistance may be an important contributor to the risk for age-related cardiovascular diseases and cancer among middle-aged, smoker men [37].

Smoking is a double-edged sword for the oropharyngeal mucosa by means of its local toxic and systemic, harmful metabolic and hormonal impacts. The carcinogenic capacity of tobacco prevails first as a local noxa in the oral cavity, and later the smoking-related unfavourable metabolic effects return by means of the circulation. However, advantageous Mediterranean dietary habits, such as high fruit, vegetable, fish and desaturated oil consumption cause a decreased cancer risk for the upper aerodigestive tract even in heavy smokers [82,123].

Alcohol Consumption, Insulin Resistance and Cancer Risk

Alcohol consumption is associated with contradictory, Janus-faced metabolic effects. Results of epidemiological studies suggest that mild to moderate alcohol intake is associated with advantageous metabolic effects, such as lower prevalence of insulin resistance, metabolic syndrome, type-2 diabetes and their cardiovascular complications [46]. In contrast, the two extremes namely complete abstinence and excessive drinking are risks for insulin resistant states [114].

Alcohol consumption has thorough influence on the metabolic processes, especially on lipids [106]. Moderate alcohol intake (<20 g/die) improves lipid profile, increases insulin sensitivity and decreases both waist circumference and serum insulin level. HDL-cholesterol level of the serum shows a parallel increase with moderate doses of alcohol intake. Serum triglyceride level shows a favorable decrease in moderate drinkers, whereas an increased level can be found in excessive drinkers. Moderate alcohol consumption has a well-known cardio-protective effect, resulting from decreased coagulation activity, improvement of dyslipidemia and antioxidant capacity with decreased lipid oxidation.

Clinical studies on middle-aged male patients justified an increased adiponectin and decreased TNF-α level in moderate drinkers, which means a decreased risk for insulin resistance [114]. Adiponectin, an adipocyte derived plasma protein has been negatively associated with adiposity and insulin resistance [39]. It seems to be an important endogenous factor, which increases the effect of insulin.

In older women, lifetime alcohol consumption was associated with type-2 diabetes in a U-shape fashion. Moderate alcohol consumption was the lowest risk for insulin resistance as compared with both excessive drinking and abstinence [13]. In postmenopausal women, with a constant body weight, moderate alcohol consumption reduces the bioavailable IGF-I level in the serum [74]. These data suggest that moderate alcohol intake may reduce the cancer risk in postmenopausal women either by the reduction of bioavailable IGF-I level or by an increased insulin sensitivity.

Regular alcohol consumption exhibits close correlation with the female sexual steroid metabolism in a dose related manner. Estrogen levels may be higher in women who regularly consume alcoholic beverages especially in postmenopausal cases [96] Alcohol mediated increase of estrogen synthesis may be attributed to an enhanced aromatase activity in the peripheral fatty tissue or to an effect on the adrenal gland [47,100]. Another supposed possibility is the decreased catabolism of sex steroids in the liver caused by a concomitant alcohol metabolism.

In clinical studies the effect of regular, moderate alcohol intake was examined on the mortality of aged women (above 55 yrs). Alcohol consumption was inversely associated with cardiovascular mortality and total mortality both in the never smoker and former smoker groups, but was not among current smokers [33]. Studies on middle-aged and elderly women indicated that moderate alcohol consumption might be associated with decreased risk of renal cell carcinoma [102]. Both increased insulin sensitivity and elevated estrogen level may explain these advantageous effects of moderate ethanol intake in postmenopausal women.

Drinking has fairly contradictory effects on the tumor genesis as well. Though moderate alcohol consumption has beneficial effect on the metabolism, some authors could not identify a threshold level of drinking below which there is no increased risk for cancer [9].

Ethanol itself has no direct carcinogenic capacity, but its metabolism leads to generation of acetaldehyde, which is mutagenic and carcinogenic through binding directly to DNA and transcription factor proteins [99]. Acetaldehyde may also be produced locally in the mouth from ethanol through bacterial oxidative metabolism [70]. This mechanism may play major role in oropharyngeal cancer initiation, especially in case of neglected oral hygiene.

Alcohol consumption is a well-known strong risk factor for oral and upper alimentary tract cancers [9,19,44] particularly if it is combined with smoking. Concentrated drinks have chronic irritant impact on the oral and pharyngeal mucosa, which results in chronic inflammation, increased regenerative processes and deliberation of free radicals and cytokines. All these changes mean risks for malignancies [128]. Excessive alcohol intake enhances the risk for cancers not only in the upper aerodigestive tract but also in the stomach, colon, rectum, liver and breast [9].

However, recent studies proved that moderate alcohol intake is not a risk factor for many of the gastrointestinal diseases, which are associated with excessive alcohol consumption [125]. Furthermore, no positive correlation was observed between alcohol consumption and cancer risk at several sites. Clinical studies did not support an association between moderate alcohol intake and cancers of the ovary, pancreas and lungs [19,48,91].

There is a wide spread conception that even light to moderate alcohol consumption has carcinogenic effect on the female breast [9,117,126]. As ethanol intake increases the endogenous sex hormone production an elevated estrogen level may be accused at least partially of its carcinogenic potential [31].

However, moderate alcohol consumption in women is strongly associated with low risk for insulin resistance and the associated cardiovascular complications [78]. A well known fact that moderate alcohol intake improves the insulin resistance, which is a high risk factor for breast cancer. Considering these correlations, tumor inducing capacity of moderate drinking would be a striking contradiction.

In France and Italy, the effect of moderate drinking and different alcoholic beverages was studied in relation to oral diseases. Moderate drinking and especially red wine showed protective effect against oral leukoplakia and oral cancer [14,98]. This favorable effect of red wine may be explained by the resveratrol content, which may contribute to the anticancer capacity at several sites. Resveratrol inhibits the metabolic activation of carcinogenic agents, has antioxidant and anti-inflammatory properties, decreases cell proliferation and induces apoptosis.

Considering the thorough metabolic effects of alcohol, excessive alcohol consumption may be a tumor risk factor by promotion of dyslipidemia, oxidative stress and insulin resistance. Currently, the correlations between moderate alcohol consumption and cancer risk are controversial and require further investigations.

Aging, Insulin Resistance and Cancer Risk

Aging is a physiological process associated with gradually decreasing insulin sensitivity. Aging thoroughly alters the mechanism of cellular metabolism growth and proliferation [122].

With age oxidative stress and non-enzymatic glycation of protein structures are enhanced, which disadvantageously alter the function, growth and proliferation of cells [54]. In aged people the genome is much more vulnerable and there are also many defects in the repair mechanisms.

Age is a predictor of a variety of diseases related to insulin resistance. Prevalence of age-related diseases increases continuously in aged patients. In a prospective study, the effect of insulin resistance was evaluated on the clinical events [38]. Type-2 diabetes, hypertension, coronary heart disease, stroke and cancer developed significantly more frequently in the most insulin resistant tertile of the cases, whereas no such events were registered in the most insulin sensitive tertile. These literary data suggest that grade of insulin resistance is a more important risk factor for age-related diseases than age among old people.

The prevalence of age-related diseases shows steep increase after menopause in women. In aged women who have not undergone HRT, every year after menopause confers a negative influence on glucose tolerance and increases the risk of insulin resistance [133]. Consequently, in women the years after menopause have stronger impact on insulin resistance and associated diseases than chronological age. Associations of sexual hormone equilibrium and insulin sensitivity are discussed in Chapter 7.

Importance of Associations between Insulin Resistance and Cancer Risk

Close correlations between insulin resistance and cancer risk supply widespread possibilities in the field of prevention and treatment of cancers.

Way of life and a healthy diet have increasingly great role in the prevention of chronic diseases and cancers. Physical activity and loss of weight may increase insulin sensitivity and at the same time decrease the risk for both cardiovascular diseases and malignancies.

Considering the correlations between insulin resistance and progression of tumors, increase in insulin sensitivity is a promising possibility for cancer treatment. Local and metastatic spread of cancers at several sites, such as breast, colon and prostate may also be beneficially influenced by a healthy lifestyle.

There are insulin-sensitizing drugs, which may arrest cancer spread by maintenance of euglycemia [69]. Decrease of oxidative stress is also beneficial to hamper tumor spread by abandonment of smoking and consumption of antioxidant vitamins.

Recently, moderate alcohol consumption seems to be more advantageous in contrast to complete abstinence as it increases insulin sensitivity, which in turn improves the life expectancy of cancer patients. Overlooked insulin resistance should be revealed and treated in patients suffering of cancer.

References

[1] Adami HO, Chow WH, Nyren O: Excess risk of primary liver cancer in patients with diabetes mellitus. *J. Natl. Cancer Inst.* 88:1472-1476, 1996

[2] Agarwall GB, Natarajan K: Tumor necrosis factors: developments during the last decade. *Eur. Cytokine Netw*. 7:93-124, 1996

[3] Allen NE, Appleby PN, Davey GK, Kaaks R, Rinaldi S, Key TJ: The Associations of diet with serum insulin-like growth factor I and its main binding proteins in 292 women: meat-eaters, vegetarians, and vegans. *Cancer Epidemiol. Biomark and Prev.* 11: 1441-1448, 2002

[4] Augustin LSA, Gallus S, Franceschi S, Negri E, Jenkins D, Kendall CWC, dal Maso L, Talamini R, La Vecchia C: Glycemic index and load and risk of upper aero-digestive tract neoplasms. *Cancer Causes and Control* 14:657-662, 2003

[5] Augustin L, Gallus S, Negri E, La Vecchia C: Glycemic index, glycemic load and risk of gastric cancer. *Ann. Oncol*, 15:581-584, 2004a

[6] Augustin LS, Galeone C, Dal Maso L, Pelucchi C, Ramazotti V, Jenkins DJ, Montella M, Talamini R, Negri E, Franceschi S, La Vecchia C: Glycemic index, glycemic load and risk of prostate cancer. *Int. J. of Cancer* 112:446-450, 2004b

[7] Balkau B, Kahn H, Courbon D, Eschwege E, Ducimetiere P: Hyperinsulinemia predicts fatal liver cancer but is inversely associated with fatal cancer at some other sites: The Paris Prospective Study. *Diabetes Care* 24: 843-849, 2001

[8] Banerjee AG, Gopalakrishnan VK, Vishwanatha JK: Inhibition of nitric oxide-induced apoptosis by nicotine in oral epithelial cells. Mol Cell Biochem, 305:113-121, 2007

[9] Bagnardi V, Blangiardo M, La Vecchia C, Corrao G: Alcohol consumption and the risk of cancer: a meta-analysis. *Alcohol Res. and Health* 25:263-270, 2001

[10] Bahar G, Feinmesser R, Shpitzer T, Popovtzer A, Nagler RM: Salivary analysis in oral cancer patients: DNA and protein oxidation, reactive nitrogen species, and antioxidant profile. *Cancer* 109:54-59, 2007

[11] Bartsch C, Bartsch H, Blask DE, Cardinali DP, Hrushesky WJM, Mecke D, editors: *The pineal gland and cancer*. Berlin, Springer, 2001

[12] Berclaz G, Li S, Price KN et al: Body mass index as a prognostic feature in operable breast cancer: The International Breast Cancer Study Group experience. *Ann. Oncol,* 15: 875-884, 2004

[13] Beulens JW, Stolk RP, van der Schouw YT, Grobbee DE, Hendriks HF, Bots ML: Alcohol consumption and risk of type 2 diabetes among older women. *Diabetes Care* 28: 2933-2938, 2005

[14] Bianchini F, Vainio H: Wine and resveratrol: mechanisms of cancer prevention (Review). *Eur. J. Cancer Prev.* 12:417-425, 2003

[15] Bloomgarden ZT: Definitions of the insulin resistace syndrome: The 1st Word Congress on the Insulin Resistance Syndrome. *Diab. Care* 27:824, 2004

[16] Bloomgarden ZT: Second World Congress on the Insulin Resistance Syndrome: Mediators, pediatric insulin resistance, the polycystic ovary syndrome, and malignancy. *Diab. Care* 28:1821-1830, 2005

[17] Bosetti C, Negri E, Franceschi S, Pelucchi C, Talamini R, Montella M, Conti E, La Vecchia C: Diet and ovarian cancer risk: a case-control study in Italy. *Int. J. Cancer*, 93:911-915, 2001

[18] Bosetti C, Gallus S, Trichopoulou A, Talamini R, Franceschi S, Negri E, La Vecchia C: Influenece of the mediterranean diet on the risk of cancers of the upper aerodigestive tract. *Cancer Epidemiol. Biomark and Prev*. 12:1091-1094, 2003

[19] Brown LM: Epidemiology of alcohol-associated cancers. Alcohol 35:161-168, 2005

[20] Burr B, Nagi D: Exercise and Sport in Diabetes.Wiely and Sons, 1999

[21] Cagnati A, Arangino S, Renzi A et al: Influence of melatonin administration on glucose tolerance and insulin sensitivity of postmenopausal women. *Clin. Endocrinol.* 54:339-346, 2001

[22] Calle EE, Kaaks R: Overweight, obesity and cancer: epidemiological evidence and proposed mechanisms. *Nat. Rev. Cancer*, 4:579-591, 2004

[23] Carboni JM, Lee AV, Hadsell DL, et al: Tumor development by transgenic expression of a constitutively active insulin-like growth factor I receptor. *Cancer Res*. 65:3781-2005

[24] Chlebowsky RT, Aiello E, McTiernan A: Weight loss in breast cancer management. *J. Clin. Oncol*. 20:1128-1143, 2002

[25] Chlebowski RT: Obesity and early-stage breast cancer. *J. Clin. Oncol*, 23:1345-1347, 2005

[26] Clandinin MT, Cheema CJ, Field ML, Garg J, Vendatraman J, Clandinin TR: Dietary fat: exogenous determination of membrane structure and cell function. *FASEB J*. 5:2761, 1991

[27] Cowey S, Hardy RW: The metabolic syndrome: A high-risk state for cancer? *Am. J. Pathol*. 169:1505-1522, 2006

[28] DeFronzo RA, Ferrannini E: Insulin resistance: a multifaceted syndrome responsible for NIDDM, obesity, hypertension, dyslipidemia and atherosclerotic cardiovascular disease. *Diabetes Care* 14:173-194, 1991

[29] Del Giudice ME, Fantus IG, Ezzat S et al: Insulin and related factors in premenopausal breast cancer risk. *Breast Cancer Res. Treat* 47:111-120, 1998

[30] Ding XZ, Feshenfeld DM, Murphy L et al: Physiological concentrations of insulin augment pancreatic cell proliferation and glucose utilization by activating MAP kinase, P13 kinase and enchancing GLUT-1 expression. *Pancreas* 21:310-320, 2000

[31] Dorgan JF, Baer DJ, Albert PS, Judd JT, Brown ED et al: Serum hormones and the alcohol-breast cancer association in postmenopausal women. *J. Natl. Cancer Inst*. 93: 710-715, 2001

[32] Duncan G, Perri M, Theriaque D et al: Exercise training, without weight loss increases insulin sensitivity and postheparin plasma lipase activity in previously sedentary adults. *Diabetes Care* 26:557-562, 2003

[33] Ebbert JO, Janney CA, Sellers TA, Folsom AR, Cerhan JR: The association of alcohol consumption with coronary heart disease mortality and cancer incidence varies by smoking history. *J. General Intern. Medicine* 20:14-20, 2005

[34] Egan BM: Insulin resistance and sympathic nervous system. *Curr. Hypertens Rep*. 5:247-254, 2003.

[35] Eliasson B, Attval S, Taskinen MR, Smith U: The insulin resistance syndrome in smokers is related to smoking habits. Arterioscler and Thromb 14:1946-1950, 1994

[36] Enger SM, Greif JM, Polikoff J et al: Body weight correlates with mortality in early stage breast cancer. *Arch Surg*. 139:954-960. 2004

[37] Facchini FS, Hollenbeck CB, Jeopesen J: Insulin resistance and cigarette smoking. *Lancet* 339:1128-1130, 1992

[38] Facchini FS, Hua N, Abbasi F et al: Insulin resistance as a predictor of age related diseases. *J. Clin. Endocrinol. and Metab*. 86:3574-3578, 2001

[39] Fasshauer M, Paschke R: Regulation adipocytokines and insulin resistance. *Diabetologia* 46:1594-1603, 2003

[40] Ferrannini E, Barrett EJ, Bevilacqua S, DeFronzo RA: Effects of fatty on glucose production and utilization in man. *J. Clin. Invest.* 72:1737, 1983

[41] Field CJ, Ryan EA, Thomson ABR, Clandinin MT: Diet fat composition alters membrane phospholipid composition, insulin binding and glucose metabolism in adipocytes from control and diabetic animals. *J. Biol. Chem.* 265:43,1990

[42] Ford ES, Giles WH, Mokdad AH: Increasing prevalence of the metabolic syndrome among U.S. adults. *Diabetes Care* 27: 2444-2449, 2004

[43] Franceschi S, Talamini R, Barra S, Baron AE, Negri E, Bidoli E et al: Smoking and drinking in relation to cancers of the oral cavity, pharynx, larynx and esophagus in Northern Italy. *Cancer Res.* 50:6502-6507, 1990

[44] Franceschi S, Bidoli E, Negri E, Barbone F, La Vecchia C: Alcohol and cancers of the upper aerodigestive tract in men and women. *Cancer Epidemiol. Biomarkers and Prev.* 4:299-304, 1994

[45] Franceschi S, Favero A, Conti E, Talamini R, Volpe R, Negri E, Barzan L, La Vecchia C: Food groups, oils and butter, and cancer of the oral cavity and pharynx. *Cancer* 80: 614-620, 1999

[46] Freiberg MS, Cabral HJ, Heeren TC, Vasan RS, Ellison RC: Alcohol consumption and the prevalence of the metabolic syndrome in the U.S. A cross-sectional analysis of data from the Third National Health and Nutrition Examination Survey. *Diabetes Care* 27: 2954-2959, 2004

[47] Gavaler JS, Van Thiel DH: The associaton between moderate alcoholic beverage consumption and serum estradiol and testosterone levels in normal postmenopausal women: relationship to the literature. *Alcohol Clin. Exp. Res.* 16:87-92, 1992

[48] Genkinger JM, Hunter DJ, Spiegelman D, Anderson KE, Buring JE, Freudenheim JL, Goldbohm RA, Harnack L, Hankinson SE, Larsson SC, Leitzmann M, McCullough ML, Marshall J, Miller AB, Rodriguez C, Rohan TE, Schatzakin A, Schouten LJ, Wolk A, Zhang SM. Smith-Warner SA: Alcohol intake and ovarien cancer risk: a pooled analysis of 10 cohort studies. *Br. J. Cancer* 94:757-762, 2006

[49] Gerlain-Biquez C, Vol S, Tichet J, Caradec A, D'Hour A, Balkau B: The metabolic syndrome in smokers: the D.E.S.I.R. study. *Diabetes Metab.* 29:226-234, 2003

[50] Giovanucci E, Pollak M, Liu Y et al: Nutritional predictors of insulin-like growth factor I and their relationships in men. *Cancer Epidemiol. Biomark and Prev.* 12:84-89, 2003

[51] Golf DC, Zaccaro DJ, Haffner SM et al: Insulin sensitivity and risk the risk of incident hypertension: insights from the insulin resistance. (Atherosclerosis Study). *Diabetes Care* 26:805-809, 2003

[52] Gupta K, Krishnaswamy G, Karnad A et al: Insulin: A novel factor in carcinogenesis. *Am. J. Med. Sci.* 323:140-145, 2002

[53] Hammarsten J, Hogstedt B: Hyperinsulinaemia: A prospectiv risk factor for lethal clinical prostate cancer. *Eur. J. Cancer* 41:2887-2895, 2005

[54] Harman D: Free radicals in aging. *Mol. Cell. Biochem.* 84:155-161, 1988

[55] Hershkovich O, Shafat I, Nagler RM: Age-related changes in salivary antioxidant profile: possible implications for oral cancer. *Journals of Gerontology Series* A-Biologocal Sciences and Medical Sciences 62:361-366, 2007

[56] Higginbotham S, Zhang ZF, Lee IM, Cook NR, Giovanucci E, Buring JE, Liu S: Dietary glycemic load and risk of colorectal cancer in the Women's Health Study. *J. Natl. Cancer Inst*, 96:229-233, 2004

[57] Hirose K, Toyama T, Iwata H et al. Insulin, insulin-like growth factor-1 and breast cancer risk in Japanese women. *Asian Pac. J. Cancer Prev.* 4:239-246, 2003

[58] Ishizaka N, Ishizaka Y, Toda E, Nagai R, Yamakado M: Association between smoking, hematological parameters, and metabolic syndrome in Japanese men. American Diabetes Association 29:741, 2006

[59] Jee SH, Ohrr H, Sull JW, YunJE, Ji M, Samet JM: Fasting serum glucose level and cancer risk in Korean men and women. *JAMA* 293:194-202, 2005

[60] Jump DB, Clarke SD, Thelen A, Liimatta M, Ren B, Badin MV: Dietary fat, genes and human health. *Adv. Experiment Med. Biol.* 422:167-176, 1997

[61] Kahn CR, Folli F: Molecular determinant of insulin action. *Hormon Res.* 39:93-101, 1993

[62] Kahn CR: Insulin receptors and insulin signalling in normal and disease states. In: Alberti KGM, Zimmet P, DeFronzo RA, Keen H, (eds): International Textbook of Diabetes mellitus. 2nd ed. pp. 437-466. John Wiley and Sons, Chichester, 1997

[63] Key TJ, Applyby PN, Reeves GK: Body mass index, serum sex hormones and breast cancer risk in postmenopausal women. *J. Natl. Cancer Inst.* 95: 1218-1226, 2003

[64] Key TJ, Schatzkin A, Willett WC, Allen NE, Spencer EA, Travis RC: Diet, nutrition and the prevention of cancer. *Public Health Nutr.* 1:187-200, 2004

[65] Kido Y, Nakae J, Accili D: Clinical review: The insulin receptor and its cellular targets. *J. Clin. Endocrinol. Metab.* 86: 972-979, 2001

[66] Kim YI: Diet, lifestyle, and colorectal cancer: is hyperinsulinemia the missing link? *Nutr. Rev.* 56:275-279, 1998

[67] Kreimer AR, Randi G, Herrero R, Castellsague X, Vecchia CL, Franceschi S: Diet and body mass, and oral and oropharyngeal squamous cell carcinomas: Analysis from the IARC multinational case controll study. *Int. J. Cancer* 118:2293-2297, 2006

[68] Kriska A, Pereira M, Hanson R et al: Association of physical activity and serum insulin concentration in two population at high risk to type 2 diabetes, but differing by BMI. *Diabetes Care* 24:1175-1180, 2001

[69] Krone CA, Ely JTA: Controlling hyperglycemia as an adjunct to cancer therapy. *Integr. Cancer Ther.* 4:25-31, 2005

[70] Kurkivuori J, Salasouro V, Kaihovaara P, Kari K, Rautemaa R, Gronroos L, Meurman JH, Salaspuro M: Acetaldehyde production from ethanol by oral streptococci. *Oral Oncology* 43:181-186, 2007

[71] Landsberg L. Insulin mediated sympathetic stimulation: role in the pathogenesis of obesity related hypertension (or how insulin affects blood pressure and why). *Hypertension* 19:523-528, 2001

[72] La Vecchia C, Chatenoud L, Altieri A, Tavani A: Nutrition and health: epidemiology of diet, cancer and cardiovascular disease in Italy. *Nutr. Met. and Cariovasc. Dis.* 11: 10-15, 2001b

[73] La Vecchia C: Mediterranean diet and cancer. (Review). *Public Health Nutr.* 7:965-968, 2004b

[74] Lavigne JA, Baer DJ, Wimbrow HH, Albert PS, Brown ED, Judd JT, Campbell WS, Giffen CA, Dorgan JF, Hartman TJ, Barrett JC, Hursting SD, Taylor PR: Effects of alcohol on insulin-like growth factor I and insulin-like growth factor binding protein 3 in postmenopausal women. *Am. J. Clin. Nutr.* 81:503-507, 2005

[75] Lehmann R, Vokoc A, Niedermenn K et al: Loss of abdominal fat improvement of cardiovascular risk profile by regular moderate exercise training in patients with NIDDM. *Diabetologia* 38:1313-1319, 1995

[76] LeRoith D, Baserga R, Helman L, et al: Insulin-like growth factors and cancer. *Ann. Intern. Med.* 122:54-59, 1995

[77] Lindblad P, Chow WH, Chan J: The role of diabetes mellitus in the etiology of renal cell cancer. *Diabetologica* 42:107-112, 1999

[78] Longnecker MP, Tseng M: Alcohol, hormones and postmenopausal women. *Alcohol Health Res. World* 22:185-189, 1998

[79] Malasanos TH, Stacpoole PW: Biological effects of ω-3 fatty acids in diabetes mellitus. *Diabetes Care* 14:1160, 1991

[80] Mangelsdorf D, Thummel C, Beatoo M et al: The nuclear receptor superfamily: the second decade. *Cell* 83:835-839, 1995

[81] Manicardi V, Camellini L, Bellodi G. et al: Evidence for an association of high blood pressure and hyperinsulinemia in obese men. *J. Clin. Endocrinol. Metab.* 62:1302-1304, 1986

[82] Marchioni DM, Fisberg RM, Francisco de Gois Filho J, Kowalski LP, Brasilino de Carvalho M, Abrahao M, Latorre Mdo R, Eluf-Neto J, Wunsch Filho V: Dietary patterns and risk of oral cancer: a case-control study in Sao Paulo, Brazil. Revista de Saude Publica 41:19-26, 2007

[83] Mattison R, Jensen M: The adipocyte as an endocrine cell. *Curr. Opin. Endocrinol. Diabetes* 10:317-321, 2003

[84] McKeown-Eyssen G: Epidemiology of colorectal cancer revisited: are serum triglycerides and plasma glucose associated with risk? *Cancer Epidemiol Biomark and Prev.* 3:687-695, 1994

[85] McLaughlin T, Abbasi F, Cheal K et al: Use of metabolic markers to identify overweight individuals who are insulin resistant. *Ann. Intern. Med.* 139:802-809, 2003

[86] McTiernan A: Associations between energy balance and body mass index and risk of breast carcinoma in a women from diverse racial and ethnic backgrounds in the U.S. cancer. *Cancer* 88:1248-1255, 2000

[87] Michels KB, Ekbom A: Caloric restriction and incidence of breast cancer. *JAMA* 291-1226-1230, 2004

[88] Morse DE, Psoter WJ, Cleveland D, Cohen D, Mohit-Tabatabai M, Kosis DL, Eisenberg E: Smoking and drinking in relation to oral cancer and oral epithelial dysplasia. *Cancer Causesand Control* 1800:919-929, 2007

[89] Muti P, Quattrin T, Grant BJB et al: Fasting glucose is a risk factor for breast cancer. *Cancer Epidemiol. Biomark and Prev.* 11:1361-1368, 2002

[90] Nilsen TI, Vatten LJ: Prospective study of colorectal cancer risk and physical activity, diabetes, blood glucose and BMI: exploring the hyperinsulinaemia hypothesis. *Br. J. Cancer* 84:417-422, 2001

[91] Nishino Y, Wakai K, Kondo T, Seki N, Ito Y, Suzuki K, Ozasa K, Watanabe Y, Ando M, Tsubono Y, Tsuji I, tamakoshi A; JACC Study Group. Alcohol consumption and lung cancer mortality in Japan collaborative cohort (JACC) study. *J. Epidemiol.* 16: 49-56, 2006
[92] Ogihara S, Yamada M, Saito T et al: Insulin potentiated mitogenic effect of epidermal growth factor on cultured guinea pig gastric mucous cells. *Am. J. Physiol.* 271:104-112, 1996
[93] Ogihara T, Asano T, Ando K et al: Insulin resistance with enhanced insulin signalling in high salt diet fed rats. *Diabetes* 50:573-583, 2001
[94] Olefsky JM: The insulin receptor: a multifunctional protein. *Diabetes* 39:1009-1016, 1990
[95] Olefsky JM: The insulin receptor: its role in insulin resistance of obestity and diabetes. *Diabetes* 25:1154-1162, 1976
[96] Onland-Moret NC, Peeters PHM, van der Schouw YT, Grobbee DE, van Gils CH: Alcohol and endogenous sex steroid levels in postmenopausal women: A cross-sectional study. *J. Clin. Endocrinol. Metab.* 90:1414-1419, 2005
[97] Pan SY, Johnson KC, Ugnat AM et al: Association of obesity and cancer risk in Canada. *Am. J. Epidemiol.* 159:259-268, 2004
[98] Petti S, Scully C: Association between different alcoholic beverages and leukoplakia among non- to moderate-drinking adults: a matched case-control study. *Eur. J. Cancer* 42:521-527, 2006
[99] Poschl G, Seitz HK: Alcohol and Cancer. Alcohol and Alcoholism. 39:155-165, 2004
[100] Purohit V: Can alcohol promote aromatization of androgens to estrogens? A review. *Alcohol* 22:123-127, 2000
[101] Rai B, Kharb S, Jain R, Anand, SC: Salivary vitamins E and C in oral cancer. *Redox Report* 12:163-164, 2007
[102] Rashidkhani B, Akesson A, Lindblad P, Wolk A: Alcohol consumption and risk of renal cell carcinoma: a prospective study of Swedish women. *Int. J. Cancer* 117:848-853, 2005
[103] Reaven GM: Banting lecture 1988: Role of insulin resistance in human disease. *Diabetes* 37:1595-1607, 1988
[104] Reaven GM: Role of insulin resistance in human disease (syndrome X): an expanded definition. *Annu. Rev.* 44:121-131, 1993
[105] Reaven GM: Insulin resistance, cardiovascular disease, and the metabolic syndrome: How well do the emperor's clothes fit? *Diabetes Care* 27:1011-1012, 2004
[106] Rimm EB, Williams P, Fosher K et al: Moderate alcohol intake and lower risk of coronary heart disease: meta-analysis of effects on lipids and hemostatic factors. *BMJ* 319:1523-1528, 1999
[107] Rogers MA, Yamamoto C, King DS et al: Improvement in glucose tolerance after 1 week of exercise in patients with mild NIDDM. *Diabetes Care* 11:613-618, 1988
[108] Rohr UD, Herold J: Melatonin deficiencies in women. *Maturitas*, 41 Suppl 1, S85-S104, 2002
[109] Rose DP: Dietary fatty acids and cancer. *Am. J. Clin. Nutr.* 66:S998-S1003, 1997

[110] Shao L, Huang Q, Luo et al: Detection of the differentielly expressed gene IGF-binding protein-related protein-1 and analysis of its relationship to fasting glucose in Chinese colorectal cancer patients. *Endocr. Relat. Cancer* 11:141-148, 2004

[111] Schneider SH, Khandadirian AK, Amorosa LF et al: Ten years experience with an exercise-based outpatient life style modification program in the treatment of diabetes mellitus. *Diabetes Care* 15:1800-1810, 1992

[112] Schoenle EJ, Zenobi PD, Torresani T, et al: Recombinant human insulin-like growth factor-I (rhIGF I) reduces hyperglycemia in patients with extreme insulin resistance. *Diabetológia* 34:675-679, 1991

[113] Slattery ML, Ballard-Barbash R, Edwards S et al:Body mass index and colon cancer: an evaluation of the modifying effects of estrogen (United States) *Cancer Causes Control* 14:75-84, 2003

[114] Sierksma A, Patel H, Ouchi N et al: Effect of moderate alcohol consumption on adiponectin, tumor necrosis factor alpha and insulin sensitivity. *Diabetes Care* 24:184-189, 2004

[115] Soler M, Chatenoud L, Negri E et al: Hypertension and hormon-related neoplasms in women. *Hypertension* 34:320-325, 1999

[116] Steinberg HO, Charker H, Leaming R et al: Obesity/insulin resistance is associated with endothel dysfunction. Implications for the syndrome of insulin resistance. *J. Clin.* Invest 97:2601-2610, 1996

[117] Stolzenberg-Solomon RZ, Chang SC, Leitzmann MF, Johnson KA, Johnson C, Buys SS, Hoover RN, Ziegler RG: Folate intake, alcohol use, and postmenopausal breast cancer risk in the Prostate, Lung, Colorectal, and Ovarian Cancer Screening Trial. *Am. J. Clin. Nutr.* 83:895-904, 2006

[118] Suba Zs, Barabás J, Takács D, Szabó Gy, Ujpál M: Epidemiological correlations of insulin resistance and salivary gland tumors. *Orvosi Hetilap* (in Hungarian) 146:1727-1732, 2005

[119] Suba Zs, Barabás J, Szabó Gy, Takács D, Ujpál M: Increased prevalence of diabetes and obesity in patients with salivary gland tumors. *Diabetes Care* 28:228, 2005

[120] Suba Zs, Ujpál M: Disorders of glucose metabolism and oral cancer risk. Fogorv Szle 100:250-257, 2007

[121] Taskinen MR: Diabetic dyslipidemia: from basic research to clinical practice. *Diabetologia* 46:733-749, 2003

[122] Tatar M, Bartke A, Antebi A: The endocrine regulation of aging by insulin like signals. *Science* 299:1346-1351, 2003

[123] Tavani A, Gallus S, La Vecchia C, Talamini R, Barbone F, Herrero R, Franceschi S: Diet and risk of oral and pharyngeal cancer. An Italian case-control study. *Eur. J. Cancer Prev.* 10:191-195, 2001

[124] Tavani A, Giordano L, Gallus S, Talamini R, Franceschi S, Giacosa A, Montella M, La Vecchia C: Consumption of sweet foods and breast cancer risk in Italy. *Annals of Oncology* 17:341-345, 2006

[125] Taylor B, Rehm J, Gmel G: Moderate alcohol consumption and the gastrointestinal tract. *Dig. Dis.* 23:170-176, 2005

[126] Terry MB, Zhang FF, Kabat G, Britton JA, Teitelbaum SL, Neugut AI, Gammon MD: Lifetime alcohol intake and breast cancer risk. *Ann. Epidemiol.* 16:230-240, 2006

[127] Tikhonoff V, Staessen JA: Hormonal regulation of human adipocytes at the cross-roads between obesity and hypertension. *J. Hypertens* 20:839-841, 2002

[128] Tsuji S, Kawai N, Tsuji M, Kawano S, Hori M. Review article: inflammation-related promotion of gastrointestinal carcinogenesis: a perigenetic pathway. *Aliment Pharmacol. Ther* .18:82-89, 2003

[129] Ujpál M, Matos O. Bíbok Gy, Somogyi A, Szabó Gy, Suba Zs: Diabetes and oral tumors in Hungary: Epidemiological correlations. *Diabetes Care* 27:770-774, 2004.

[130] Voskuil DW, Vrieling A, van't Veer LJ, Kampman E, Rookus MA: The insulin-like growth factor system in cancer prevention: potential of dietary intervention strategies. *Cancer Epidemiol. Biomark and Prev.* 14:195-203, 2005

[131] Welsch CW: Dietary fat, calories and experimental mammary gland tumorigenesis. *Cancer Res.* 52:S2040, 1992

[132] Werner H, Katz J: The emerging role of insulin-like growth factors in oral biology (Review). *J. Dental Res.* 83:832-836, 2004

[133] Wu ShI, Chou P, Tsai ShT: The impact of years since menopause on the development of impaired glucose tolerance. *J. Clin. Epidemiol.* 54:117-120, 2001

[134] Xu J, Huang H, Pan C, Zhang B, Liu X, Zhang L: Nicotine inhibits apoptosis induced by cisplatin in human oral cancer cell. *International Journal of Oral and Maxillofacial Surgery* 36:739-744, 2007

[135] Yeung NG, Husain I, Waterfall N: Diabetes mellitus and bladder cancer. An epidemiological relationship? *Pathol. Oncol. Res.* 9: 30-31, 2003

[136] Yu H, Rohan T et al. Role of the insulin-like growth factor family in cancer development and progression. *J. Natl. Cancer Inst.* 92:1472-89, 2000

[137] Zimmet PZ: Hyperinsulinemia - how innocent a bystander? *Diabetes Care* 16:56-69, 1993

Chapter 3

Hyperglycemia, Type-2 Diabetes and Cancer Risk

Delicacy for Cancer Cells

In the uncompensated phase of insulin resistance the secretor capacity of the insular β-cells becomes exhausted and the serum insulin level is not enough to maintain euglycemia. The increased plasma glucose level results in type-2 diabetes, which is a complex metabolic disorder with alterations of glucose, lipid, protein and nucleic acid metabolism and leads to increased cancer risk (see Chapter 2).

Type-2 diabetes is characterized mainly by disrupted glucose homeostasis with deleterious consequences to many organs and, when untreated, is associated with highly increased mortality. The etiologic factors of type-2 diabetes are combined environmental and genetic ones [3].

Prevalence of diabetes is widespread and increases continuously in the economically developed countries [86]. Obesity, population aging and urbanization are among the main causes of this increase. Nowadays, it is the seventh leading cause of death in the United States, and is a major contributor to hypertension, stroke, cardiovascular disease, blindness, kidney failure, and limb amputations, even malignancies. Unfortunately, the development of this illness is insidious, 40 to 50% of individuals with diabetes are unaware of their disease and it remains undiagnosed for a long time.

Type-2 diabetes has thorough influences on oral structures with widely varying clinical presentations and degrees of the effects [52]. As diabetes is associated with oral cancer and the expected prevalence of it is over 9% by 2025, the impact of diabetes on oral health will further increase in the future [4].

Hyperglycemia and cancer risk

Hyperglycemia promotes the neoplastic cell proliferation by several pathways. Elevated serum glucose level may play a direct role in the development of cancer by favoring the selection of malignant clones [85]. Neoplastic cells have been shown to extensively use glucose for their proliferation. Excessive glucose supply may play a pivotal role in the pentose phosphate metabolic pathway, which is characteristic for malignant cells and helps their unrestrained DNA synthesis [22].

Elevated serum glucose level has also indirect carcinogenic capacities. In diabetes mellitus the oxidation equilibrium breaks down. The elevated serum glucose concentration provokes glucose auto-oxidation and excessive formation of free radicals and glycated proteins. Decreased activities of the antioxidant scavengers and enzymes result in oxidative stress [2,69,84], which cause derangement both of DNA and the enzymes playing important role in repair mechanisms [2,11]. These noxious processes may cause severe damages in the biological structures even at a molecular level [11] and may promote gene regulation disorders leading to carcinogenesis [6,36,53]. Moreover, the oxidative stress may deteriorate the insulin resistance of diabetic patients at the receptor level [79].

Antioxidant nutrients may be utilized to prevent oral cancer as they counteract free radical-mediated cell proliferation disturbances [63]. New insights into the correlations between oxidative stress and diabetic complications may lead to a causal antioxidant therapy.

Expression of Glucose Transporters (GLUTs) and Oral Cancer Risk

Hyperglycemia leads to uncontrolled glucose transport into the cells. Insulin overproduction in insulin resistance stimulates cellular glucose uptake by inducing the overexpression of a protein family called glucose transporters [17]. These proteins are integrant components of the cell membrane and their function is the active transport of the glucose molecule through the double lipid layer [44].

GLUT4 is the only isoform of these proteins that responds adequately to insulin and constitutes the rate limitation of insulin-induced glucose uptake. In hyperglycemia GLUT1, which is another member of this glucose transporter family, shows enhanced expression and activity, which results in uncontrolled glucose transport through the cell membrane [29].

High expression of GLUT1 and its excessive glucose transporter activity is an important contributing factor to tissue injury in patients with diabetes. Recent literary results support that increased GLUT1 expression has crucial correlation with human malignancies. Higher GLUT-1 expression leads to higher intracellular glucose concentration, which favors for growth and proliferation of cancer cells [46].

Increased GLUT1 expression and progression of oral cancer show close correlations [46,59]

Non-enzymatic Glycation of Different Structures in type-2 Diabetes and Oral Cancer Risk

Sustained hyperglycemia is in correlation not only with glucose metabolism but also with alterations in lipid metabolism as well as non-enzymatic glycation of proteins, such as collagens [65]. These changes affect the function of the cell membranes and their receptor proteins and cause thorough changes in cell-cell and cell-matrix interactions [52]. Glycated products alter the vessel walls and basement membranes, which will disturb the normal oxygen and metabolite exchange [71,84].

Non-enzymatic glycation of proteins, lipids and nucleic acids in diabetic patients causes serious complications [15]. Glycated proteins, known as advanced glycation end-products (AGEs) may be formed both in diabetic and non-diabetic cases, however, their accumulation is greatly increased in diabetic patients with sustained hyperglycemia [71].

AGEs in patients with hyperglycemia have major effects at cellular level. A receptor for AGEs known as RAGE (receptor for AGE) has been identified on the surface of many cell types (endothelial cells, smooth muscle cells, monocytes/macrophages etc.), which have important role in oral and periodontal health and disease [72].

Vascular complications are classically associated both with type-2 diabetes and the earlier phases of glucose metabolism disorders. AGE deposition increases the capillary basement membrane thickness resulting in a serious narrowing of the lumen and impairs the exchange of oxygen and metabolic waste products through the capillary wall [49].

AGEs provoke also macrovascular complications. They increase the cross-link of collagen and the highly stable collagen macromolecules are resistant to normal enzymatic degradation and tissue turnover [56]. AGE-modified collagen deposits thicken the vessel wall and covalently cross-link with circulating low-density lipoprotein, contributing to development of atherosclerosis. The cumulative effects of these vascular alterations increase progressive narrowing of the vessel lumen and thrombotic obliteration and decrease the perfusion of the affected tissue. Hypoxia is advantageous for tumor cell multiplication as non-oxidative steps in the anabolic pathways characterize their metabolism.

The highly stable collagen accumulates also in the *basement membrane* of the squamous epithelial layer, altering the normal homeostatic transport. Defective transport of oxygen and other metabolites is advantageous also for malignant transformation of the epithelial layer.

Overexpression of Matrix Metalloproteinases and Oral Cancer Risk

Matrix metalloproteinases (MMPs) or collagenases are involved in remodeling of the extracellular matrix by means of their digesting capacity. This function is integrated into normal tissue growth and regeneration. Collagenase production is regulated at gene transcription level, and its expression is differentially affected by several growth factors [21].

It is a well-known fact that matrix collagenase production is increased in diabetes mellitus, which is harmful for periodontal integrity and wound healing [66]. Tetracyclines and their chemically modified variants without antibacterial effect have been shown to significantly decrease collagenase production [31]. These modified tetracyclines have potential benefits in inhibition of onset and progression of periodontal inflammation in patients with type-2 diabetes [7,28].

Excessive tissular collagenase activity in diabetes results in loosening and disintegration of the extracellular matrix, increased degradation of instable newly formed collagen and disintegration of the basement membrane. Leakages in the basement membrane promote tumor cell invasion of the underlying connective tissue, which is recognized as a fundamental step in the development of invasive epithelial cancers [25].

MMP-1 is a potent interstitial collagenase with frequently increased activity in the majority of oral dysplasias as well as in oral squamous cell cancers. Increased MMP-1 mRNA expression has been shown not only in the epithelial tumor cells but also in the fibrous connective tissue adjacent to the tumor [62]. Proteolytic enzymes released by the tumor cells catalyse breakdown of the collagen rich connective tissue barriers, which results in an aggressive local tumor invasion and metastatic spread [16]. Recent data support that overexpression of MMP-9 mRNA may be markers of malignant transformation of oral epithelial dysplasia to oral cancer [40].

Altered Inflammatory Reactions in Type-2 Diabetes and Oral Cancer Risk

Altered inflammatory reactions and immunologic responses in type-2 diabetes enhance the inclination to severe infections and malignancies at several sites. Type-2 diabetes has long been considered to have thorough influence on intraoral structures. It may seriously alter saliva secretion, mucosal health, integrity of periodontal tissues, wound healing and bone turnover rate [26,52].

Poor glycemic control is usually associated with xerostomia and sialoadenosis of the salivary glands, which includes enlargement of glandular volume and defective saliva secretion [26,74]. Decreased salivary flow may result in retrograde bacterial infection through the duct system. In patients with diabetes, an increased prevalence of salivary gland tumors may also be observed [76].

The altered host inflammatory response to *bacterial challenge* in patients with diabetes may be one of the possible explanations for the increased prevalence and severity of plaque induced gingivitis and periodontitis. Though periodontitis in diabetic patients is regarded mainly as inflammation caused by bacteria, the metabolic and hormonal alterations in type-2 diabetes are also promoting factors [52].

Chronic intraoral infections in type-2 diabetes may play either direct or indirect role in cancer initiation [37,48]. Microorganisms in the dental plaque and their endotoxins have toxic effects on the neighbouring cells and may directly induce mutations in the tumor suppressor genes and protooncogenes. Furthermore, plaque bacteria may also alter the signaling pathways that affect increased proliferation and survival of the epithelial cells [78].

Destructive gingivitis and periodontitis in patients with diabetes provoke a chronic release of inflammatory cytokines, chemokines, prostaglandins, growth factors and enzymes. Chronic infections induce deliberation of reactive oxygen species, nitrogen species, lipids and further metabolites, which may act as endogenous mutagens. All of these inflammatory products are associated with disturbance of epithelial turnover [37,41]. Nowadays, chronic inflammations have been regarded as tumor promoters in the process of cancer induction [9,61]. Recent studies confirmed the suspicion that plaque induced chronic periodontitis might in fact be associated with oral cancer risk independent of smoking [78]. These correlations justify the clinical observations that plaque retention and poor oral hygiene are risk factors for oral cancer [8,68].

Type-2 diabetes is a crucial risk factor for *fungal infections*. First of all candidiasis may show an increased incidence on the vulnerable, dry mucosal surfaces. Multivariate regression analysis revealed the presence of Candida albicans hyphae to be significantly related to poor glycemic control [32]. Candida infections are especially frequent in aged, edentulous patients. Denture stomatitis, angular cheilitis and palatal papillomatosis are the most frequent manifestations. Literary data support the role of Candida albicans infection in the malignization of oral precancerous lesions, especially in case of chronic hypertrophic types in the forward position of the buccal mucosa [20].

Recent evidences suggest that viruses; such as *human papilloma virus* (HPV) also have a synergistic role in oral carcinogenesis [27]. Chronic inflammatory proliferation and ulceration of the pocket epithelium in bacterial periodontitis of patients with type-2 diabetes may be advantageous for entrance, persistence and proliferation of HPV [78].

Altered Immunologic Reactions in type-2 Diabetes

Uncontrolled hyperglycemia increases the expression of receptors for AGEs and promotes AGE-RAGE interactions. Such interactions provoke thorough changes on monocyte/macrophage membranes, induce enhanced cellular oxidative stress and activate transcription factors [83]. These signals alter the monocyte/macrophage phenotype and result in increased production of inflammatory cytokines and growth factors [43,72]. These mediators may contribute not only to the chronic inflammatory processes but also to the development of malignancies [78,80].

RAGE expression and AGE-RAGE interaction are newly recognized factors regulating cancer cell invasion. RAGE expression appears to be closely associated with the invasiveness and metastatic capacity of oral carcinoma [12,70].

The polymorphonuclear leukocytes of the dentogingival sulcus also play a major role in the maintenance of periodontal health. Numerous studies related to diabetes mellitus have shown a reduction in leukocyte function, including chemotactic responses, adherence and phagocytosis [50]. Diminished polymorphonuclear leukocyte function and persistence of bacterial challenge might then be met an elevated monocyte/macrophage response, resulting in increased tissue destruction [51].

In patients with diabetes, T-cell functions as well as cellular immune response are also impaired [73]. This diminished immune reactivity may also facilitate malignant transformation.

Considering the well-known oral manifestations of type-2 diabetes, both chronic inflammatory processes (gingivitis, periodontitis, mucositis) and atrophic epithelial lesions (cheilitis, glossitis) may be possible precursors of the malignant transformation.

Type-2 Diabetes and Risk for Oral Precancerous Lesions

The healthy oral epithelial layer is regarded as a protective barrier against toxic and carcinogenic compounds. In diabetic cases, the atrophied oral mucosa, decreased rate of salivary secretion and low salivary pH increase the development of oral lesions [26]. Atrophy, inflammation and regenerative processes may increase the permeability of the oral mucosa to carcinogens [5] and at the same time may disturb the regulation of cell proliferation as well.

Recent epidemiological studies conducted in Hungary [81] and in India [24] showed an increased prevalence of oral premalignant lesions among patients with type-2 diabetes. Earlier investigations have shown an increased prevalence of leukoplakia and lichen planus among insulin dependent (type-1) diabetic patients [1]. However, recent studies have strengthened that both precancerous and malignant oral lesions are preferentially associated with type-2 diabetes [5,81]. However, correlations between diabetes and malignization of leukoplakia were not supported by histological diagnosis till now, so informations about dysplastic features of premalignant lesions in diabetes are completely missing.

There is a gender-related difference in all cause and cardiovascular mortality related to hyperglycemia [35]. Preferential risk of women for oral premalignant lesions was also observed among patients with type-2 diabetes in several studies. Associations of premalignant oral lesions, such as oral leukoplakia, erythroplakia and submucous fibrosis with diabetes mellitus have been studied in a case control study in India [24]. Separate examinations on male and female cases resulted in striking gender related differences. A close correlation between diabetes and incidence of premalignant oral lesions among women was observed. However, no statistically significant association between diabetes mellitus and oral precancerous lesions was found in men. These differences suggest some hormonal involvement in the risk for oral precancerous lesions in women.

Clinical risk factors for oral leukoplakia have been studied in a representative sample of US population [23]. Tobacco smoking was found as the strongest, independent risk factor for oral premalignancies. Furthermore, diabetes, age and socio-economic status were also found as independent predictors of oral leukoplakia. Alcohol consumption, ethnicity, education and body mass index (BMI) showed no independent association with leukoplakia. In female cases with a history of postmenopausal estrogen replacement therapy a significantly decreased prevalence of oral leukoplakia was observed. In conclusion, this representative study justified that diabetes has a direct, and estrogen treatment an inverse association with the pathogenesis of this oral premalignancy.

Oral erythroplakia is a rare, potentially malignant lesion of the oral mucosa. A range of prevalences between 0.02% and 0.83% from different geographical areas has been documented [67]. Our working group revealed an epidemiological correlation between type-2 diabetes and increased prevalence of oral erythroplakia [81].

Type-2 Diabetes and Cancer Risk

Nowadays, type-2 diabetes is considered as a high-risk state for cancers at several sites, and this relationship should be systematically explored across further types of cancers (see Chapter 2).

Associations between diabetes and cancer risk for all and specific sites were studied among Japanese men and women [47]. Diabetes was strongly associated with cancer risk at several sites both among men and women and the authors established that diabetes might be correlated with the etiology of cancer development. Elevated fasting blood glucose and cancer risk was studied in Austria [64] and in Korea among men and women [38]. High fasting serum glucose levels and diabetes were independent risk factors for several major cancers, and the risk tended to be increased parallel with elevated fasting glucose level.

A prospective study on associations between hyperglycemia and cancer risk was performed in Sweden [75]. The association of elevated fasting glucose with total cancer risk was stronger in women as compared with men, and provided further evidence for a gender related association between abnormal glucose metabolism and cancer. Our working group in Hungary also revealed a significant correlation between elevated fasting glucose level and oral cancer risk among women but not among men (see Chapter 5).

Associations between diabetes and cancer risk were also observed in animal experiments. An accelerated tumor formation was registered in fatless mouse with type-2 diabetes and inflammation [58]. Increased risk for oral cancer in diabetic rats was attributed to the altered insulin receptor substrate-1 and focal adhesion kinase pathways [30].

Epidemiological Associations of Diabetes Mellitus and Risk for Oral Cancer in Hungary

Our working group examined the correlations between diabetes mellitus (DM) and oral premalignancies and cancers in a clinical case-control study on a pooled population of male and female cases [77,81].

The first part of the study was a *stomato-oncological screening on 200 diabetic patients* in the Medical Departments of the Semmelweis University in Budapest. The control group included 280 adult dentistry outpatients. Both inpatients and outpatients were involved into the study: 82 patients had type-1 diabetes (DM1), and 118 had type-2 diabetes (DM2). A total of 131 cases were women, and 69 were men. The average age of the patients was 45.8 years. The mean age of the patients was 36.3 years in the DM1 group, and 55.3 years in the DM2 group. The control group comprised 280 adult, otherwise healthy dentistry outpatients (109 men, 171 women) with a mean age of 47.2 years.

Two physicians performed the examinations and the data were recorded on a specially prepared questionnaire. Besides the relevant personal data, recorded information on laboratory values related to previous treatment of DM, possible complications, as well as smoking habits were also included.

Clinical examination was performed, including a thorough examination of the oral cavity and bimanual palpation of the cervical region. The examiners were not aware of the patients' diabetic state.

The results of the *stomato-oncological screening of DM patients* are presented in Table 1. The lesions found were classified into three groups: 1) inflammatory lesions, such as cheilitis and glossitis, 2) benign tissue accumulations, and 3) precancerous lesions, such as leukoplakia and erythroplakia. Malignant lesions were found neither among the 200 diabetic patients nor in the control group.

Oral cavity lesions were found in 51.5% of the DM patients. In both types of DM cases, inflammations occurred most frequently, which were followed by benign tumors, and then by precancerous lesions. In the control group, the frequency of all kinds of lesions was significantly lower ($p<0.01$).

The proportion of inflammatory lesions, benign tissue proliferations and precancerous lesions was higher among patients with DM2 than among those with DM1 (Table 3.1). The 11% incidence of leukoplakia in the DM2 group was noteworthy. The proportion of active smokers and of those who had given up smoking in this group were 38% and 32%, respectively, i.e., a total of 70% of the patients still were or had been smokers.

The second part of the study was a *retrospective DM screening of cases with oral cancer (OC).* The study comprised 610 inpatients with histologically confirmed squamous cell OC in the Department of Oral and Maxillofacial Surgery of Semmelweis University. The control group included 574 complaint- and tumor-free adults. Ratio of smokers and fasting blood glucose levels were determined in both groups, and the tumor location was registered in the cancer patients. Fasting blood glucose levels were determined repeatedly within 4 days, regarded as elevated only if it was found repeatedly high. Based on the findings, the patients were classified into three groups: 1) patients with a normal fasting blood glucose level (<6.0 mmol/1), 2) patients with an elevated fasting blood glucose (EFG) level (6.0-6.9 mmol/1), and 3) patients with DM (>6.9 mmol/1). Smoking habits in both cancer and control groups, and tumor locations in the OC group were also registered.

Diabetes screening of patients with OC and their controls resulted in conspicuous differences. Of patients with oral cancer, 14,6% had DM, whereas 9.7% displayed an elevated fasting blood glucose level, i.e., overall, 24.3% of the patients had abnormal glucose metabolism. Seventy-two of the DM patients were known cases, whereas 17 (2.8%) of them were newly diagnosed.

In the control group there were significantly fewer DM and elevated fasting glucose level cases, 5.6 and 5.5%, respectively ($p<0.01$). The distribution of malignant tumors in the oral cavity according to location for all of the patients and for the DM group is shown in Table 3.2. The most frequent OC locations among non-DM patients were the sublingual region (29%) followed by the tongue (24%). However, there were significantly more gingival and lip cancers in the DM group than in the control group ($p<0.01$).

Correlations between Diabetes and Risk of Oral Premalignant and Malignant Lesions

Our stomato-oncological screening study clarified a higher incidence of benign tumors and precancerous lesions in DM patients as compared with their controls. Our examinations revealed a higher incidence of benign tumors than reported by other authors. Bánóczy et al. found a frequency of 3,7% for the most common benign oral lesions in DM patients [10]. This was substantially lower than the 14,5% among our DM patients (10,9% for DM1, and 16,9% for DM2 patients).

Albrecht et al. found leukoplakia in 6,2% of their DM patients [1], whereas in our study, an incidence rate of 6% for leukoplakia in DM patients was observed. Of the 16 newly detected precancerous lesions that were screened out, 4 proved to be erythroplakia, i.e. 2% of the 200 diabetes patients. This is markedly higher than the literature value of 0,1% [24].

Table 3.1. Distribution of oral lesions by type and sex in the groups of the type-1 and type-2 DM

Number of cases	Control group				Type 1 DM group				Type 2 DM group			
	Men	Women	Total	%	Men	Women	Total	%	Men	Women	Total	%
All			280	100			82	100			118	100
Cheilitis, glossitis	11	15	26	9.2	6	15	21	25.6	12	25	37	31.3
Benign tumor	8	10	18	6.4	2	7	9	10.9	6	14	20	16.3
Precancerous lesions	4	5	9	3.2	2	1	3	3.6	4	9	13	11.0
Total	23	30	53	18.8	10	23	33	40.2	48	48	70	59.2

Table 3.2. Occurrence of oral cavity cancers among DM and non-DM patients

Group of patients	Location of oral cavity cancers						
	Labial	Lingual	Sublingual	Gingival	Buccal	Other	Total
Non-DM patients	73 (14%)	100 (19%)	146 (28%)	83 (16%)	21 (4%)	98 (19%)	521 (100%)
DM patients	21 (24%)	16 (18%)	13 (15%)	26 (29%)	3 (3%)	10 (11%)	89 (100%)
Total	94	116	159	109	24	108	610
Date are n (%)							

The incidence of both precancerous lesions (leukoplakia and erythroplakia) was 8% in our DM patients: 3,6% in the DM1 and 11% in the DM2 group. This value is essentially higher than the data of other Hungarian authors, who screened the general population for premalignant lesions [10]. A remarkable finding is the significantly higher incidence of leukoplakia among patients with DM2 as compared with DM1 cases.

Our study confirmed the well-known fact that smoking is a deciding risk factor for precancerous oral lesions [23,39,57]. Seventy percent of our DM patients with leukoplakia were or had been smokers. The incidence of 16,6% for premalignant lesions (leukoplakia and erythroplakia) in the smoker OC group was extraordinarily high as compared with the data of Albrecht et al. They reported an incidence of 11,5% for leukoplakia among smoking DM patients [1]. It may be stated that smoking and DM together are high-risks from the aspect of oral premalignancies.

The other aspect of our study was the DM screening of 610 inpatients with oral squamous cell carcinoma. There were significantly more patients with an abnormal glucose metabolism (DM+EFG) in the tumor group (24,3%) than in the control group (11,1%) ($p< 0.01$). Among the 89 OC patients with manifest diabetes, DM2 was predominant (97%).

The incidence of oral premalignancies and malignant tumors is higher in persons of disadvantageous social status, as these persons are also more likely to have undiagnosed or insufficiently treated DM [34]. Inadequate dental state, poor oral hygiene and certain dietary factors are also independent risk factors for OC [68], which may be fairly deteriorated by DM.

As concerns the location of oral malignancies, in the non-DM group, sublingual and lingual tumors were predominant. In the DM group, the most frequent cancer locations were the gingiva and the lower lip, which are preferentially affected by atrophic and inflammatory lesions in DM patients.

Oral precancerous lesions and tumors were more frequent among DM2 cases as compared with DM1 patients. A possible etiological factor may be the insulin resistance, the decreased sensitivity of peripheral tissues to insulin [13]. DM2 may be associated not only with hyperglycemia but also with hyperinsulinemia and elevated IGF levels, which are also regarded as high risk factors for cancer (see Chapter 2). Another important fact is that DM2 cases are generally diagnosed and treated after a longer delay, as the complaint-free latency period can take several years [26]. This period of subclinical diabetes may be advantageous for the insidious development of oral lesions.

Insulin resistance is a proven risk factor for cancers at many sites (see Chapter 2) and our findings revealed that it has a predictive role in the development of oral cavity cancers as well.

Correlations of Type-2 Diabetes and Progression of Oral Cancer

Poor prognosis of prostate, breast and colorectal cancer cases has been associated with type-2 diabetes from the late 90th [18,33,54]. Recently, impact of insulin resistance and diabetes on the outcome of all cancer has been investigated in several populations.

A Korean study justified that smoking, alcohol consumption, obesity and insulin resistance had a statistically significant, unfavorable effect on survival among male cancer patients [60]. In the United States the impact of diabetes mellitus on outcome in patients with colon cancer was examined. Diabetic patients with high risk-stage colon cancer experienced a significantly higher rate of overall mortality and cancer recurrence, even after adjustment for other predictors of colon cancer outcome [54].

Antidiabetic therapy may also influence cancer-related mortality. Patients with type-2 diabetes exposed to sulfonylureas and exogenous insulin had a significantly increased risk of cancer related mortality as compared with patients treated with insulin sensitizing Metformin [14].

Although type-2 diabetes and oral cancer are major health problems affecting the adult population in western countries, few studies have directly addressed the relationship between the two diseases or the impact of type-2 diabetes on oral cancer outcome [23,24]. The question arose as to what extent could the metabolic disturbance of diabetes influence the progression of oral cancer.

Our study was a prospective comparative examination involving a homogeneous control group, to determine the rate of progression of gingival cancers in patients with type-2 diabetes and in patients with normal glucose metabolism [82]. Gingival tumors were chosen, as our earlier investigations revealed the primacy of this location of oral cancers among diabetic patients.

A prospective follow-up study involved patients with gingival squamous cell carcinomas in stage T2-3N0M0. Their treatment comprised surgical tumor extirpation, block resection of the mandible, functional cervical dissection and 60 Gy of adjuvant irradiation. The patients were divided into a group with type-2 diabetes and a non-diabetic, control group. Cancer progression data were recorded after a 2-year period of clinical follow-up. Surgical samples were assessed histopathologically from the aspect of local and metastatic tumor spread [87].

The randomized prospective study included 100 cancer patients: 48 were allocated to the type-2 diabetes group, and 52 to the non diabetic control group. The mean age of the patients in the type-2 diabetes group was 55,8 years, while that in the control group was 57,0 years. The male:female ratio was 24:24 in the type-2 diabetes group, and 27:25 in the control group.

A total of 33% of the type-2 diabetes group and 69% of the control group were active smokers; 21% of the type-2 diabetes group and 1% of the control group had smoked previously.

Table 3.3. Distribution of progression events in the DM2 group and the control group after a 2-year follow-up period

Progression	DM2 group (n=48)	Control group (n=52)
Rate of tumor progression	30 (62,5%)	24 (46,1%)
Local recurrence	6 (12.5%)	14 (26.9%)
Local recurrence + regional metastases	24 (50%)	6 (11.5%)
Local recurrence + regional metastases + lung metastases	-	2 (3.8%)
Regional metastases	-	2 (3.8%)
Rate of death	24 (50%)	6 (11.5%)

Table 3.4. Histological degree of tumor invasion in the DM2 and control groups

Degree of tumor invasion	DM2 group (n=48)	Control group (n=52)
1.	4 (8.3%)	10 (19.2%)
2.	10 (20.8%)	27 (51.9%)
3.	14 (29.2%)	9 (17.3%)
4.	20 (41.7%)	6 (11.5%)

The distribution of tumor progression events in the diabetic and control groups of gingival cancer cases is summarized in Table 3.3.

In the type-2 diabetes group, progression was observed in 30 of the 48 cases (62,5%); 6 cases involved local recurrence (12.5%) 24 cases both local recurrence and cervical lymph node metastases (50.0%). By the end of the 2-year follow-up period, 24 of the 48 patients (50%) had died.

In the control group, 24 of the 52 patients displayed cancer progression (46,1%). Fourteen cases of them suffered of local recurrences alone (26.9%), 6 exhibited the combined occurrence of local recurrence and regional lymph node metastases, whereas in 2 cases only regional lymph node metastases were diagnosed. In 2 cases there was a combination of local recurrence, cervical and pulmonary metastases. During the 2-year follow-up period, 6 of the 52 patients (11%) had died.

Though the rate of local recurrences was higher in the control group, there were significantly more metastatic cases ($p<0.05$) and deaths ($p<0.001$) in the type-2 diabetes group during the 2-year follow-up period.

The histological results revealed a more aggressive tumor invasion in the type-2 diabetes group as compared with the control group (Table 4); the difference between the two groups was significant ($p<.01$).

Among the gingival cancer cases with type-2 diabetes grade-3 and grade-4 tumor invasion occurred more frequently; in 34 of the 48 cases (70.1%), whereas grade-1 and grade-2 invasions were characteristic in the control group; in 37 of the 52 cases (71.2%).

Type-2 Diabetes and Prognosis of Oral Cancer

Oral cancer has a poor prognosis, with a 5-year survival rate of 50% to 55% [20,57]. Local recurrence typically occurs relatively early, most often within 1 to 2 years. As tumor progression is considerably influenced by TNM stage, our cases were homogenized, and only cases with T2-T3 stages were included.

Presumably, the more rapid tumor progression in type-2 diabetes may be caused by different factors [60]. Elevated matrix metalloproteinase level and increased RAGE expression in type-2 diabetes may play an important role in both direct and metastatic spread of oral cancers [12,16]. In clinical studies increased expression of matrix metalloproteinase-2 predicted poor prognosis in squamous cell carcinoma of the tongue [88].

In diabetes mellitus the excessive glucose supply in the serum provokes an increased Glut-1 expression and glucose transport activity as compared with physiologic glucose concentrations [55]. Glut-1 has an important correlation with human malignancies. In oral cancer cases, a significant relationship between disease-related death and Glut-1 expression was observed; a high Glut-1 level predicted shorter survival [46,59].

Smoking has well-known harmful effects in terms of both oral cancer and type-2 diabetes [39,42]. In our study, the percentage of smokers was lower in the group of patients with diabetes than in the control group. This suggests that in our gingival cancer cases diabetic tissue derangement seemed to be a stronger risk factor than smoking for the progression of oral cancer.

The literary data and our results on gingival cancer cases supported the strong association of type-2 diabetes with increased spread of cancer. Patients with gingival cancer and type-2 diabetes exhibited a higher rate of metastatic lesions and of overall mortality as compared with their controls. These results permit an assumption that type-2 diabetes may be considered as a prognostic factor in cases of gingival cancer, suggesting an unfavorable course.

In patients with breast cancer the tumor progression could be hampered by physical activity, weight loss and maintenance of euglycemia [18,19]. Literary data support that a strict control of hyperglycemia may be regarded as an adjunct to cancer therapy [45]. The associations between type-2 diabetes and invasiveness of oral malignancies reveal new possibilities in the treatment and follow up of oral cancer cases. Clearing up the undiagnosed disorders of glucose metabolism in patients with oral cancer, control and correction of the metabolic parameters may improve the poor results, which have been achieved in this field till now.

References

[1] Albrecht M, Bánóczy J, Dinya E, Tamás G: Occurrence of oral leukoplakia and lichen planus in diabetes mellitus. *J. Oral Pathol. Med.* 21:364-366,1992

[2] Altmore E, Vendemiale G, Chicco D et al: Increased lipid peroxidation in type 2 poorly controlled diabetic patient. *Diabetes Metab.* 18:264-271, 1992

[3] American Diabetes association. Report of the expert committee on the diagnosis and classification of diabetes mellitus. *Diabetes Care*, 24(suppl 1):S5-S20, 2001a

[4] American diabetes association. Position statement: screening for diabetes. *Diabetes Care* 24(suppl 1):S21-S24, 2001

[5] Auluck A: Diabetes mellitus: an emerging risk factor for oral cancer? J Can Dent Assoc 73:501-503, 2007

[6] Bahar G, Feinmesser R, Shpitzer T, Popovtzer A, Nagler RM: Salivary analysis in oral cancer patients: DNA and protein oxidation, reactive nitrogen species, and antioxidant profile. *Cancer* 109:54-59, 2007

[7] Bain S, Ramamurthy NS, Impeduglia T, Scolman S, Golub LM. Rubin C: Tetracycline prevents cancellous bone loss and maintains near-normal rates of bone formation in streptozotocin diabetic rats. *Bone* 21:147-153, 1997.

[8] Balaram P, Sridhar H, Rajkumar T, Vaccarella S, Herrero R, Nandakumar A, Ravichandran K, Ramdas K, Sankaranarayanan R, Gajalakshmi V, Munoz N, Franceschi S: Oral cancer in southern India: the influence of smoking, drinking, paan-chewing and oral hygiene. *Int. J. Cancer* 98:440-445, 2002

[9] Balkwill F, Mantovani A: Inflammation and cancer: back to Wirchow? *Lancet* 57:539-545, 2001

[10] Bánóczy J, Bako A, Dombi C, Ember I, Kosa Z, Sandor J, Szabo G: Stomatooncological screening examinations: possibilities for early diagnosis. *Magy Onkol.* 45:143-148, 2001

[11] Baynes JW, Thorpe SR: Role of oxidative stress in diabetic complications: a new perspective on an old paradigm. *Diabetes* 48:1-9, 1999

[12] Bhawal UK, Ozaki Y, Nishimura M: Association of expression of receptor for advanced glycation end products and invasive activity of oral squamous cell carcinoma. *Oncology* 69:246-255, 2005

[13] Bloomgarden ZT: Definitions of the insulin resistace syndrome: The 1st Word Congress on the Insulin Resistance Syndrome. *Diabetes Care* 27:824, 2004

[14] Bowker SL, Majumdar SR, Veugelers P, Johnson JA: Increased cancer-related mortality for patients with type 2 diabetes who use sulfonylureas or insulin. *Diabetes Care* 29:254-258, 2006

[15] Brownlee M: Glycation and diabetic complications. *Diabetes* 43:836-841, 1994.

[16] Chambers AF, Matrisian LM: Changing views of the role of matrix metalloproteinases in metastasis. *J. Natl. Cancer Inst.* 89:1260-1270, 1997

[17] Charron MJ, Lodish HF: Molecular physiology of glucose transporters. *Diabetes Care* 13:209-218, 1990

[18] Chlebowsky RT, Aiello E, McTiernan A: Weight loss in breast cancer management. *J. Clin. Oncol.* 20:1128-1143, 2002

[19] Chlebowski RT: Obesity and Early-stage Breast Cancer. *J. Clin. Oncol.* 23:1345-1347, 2005

[20] Clayman, L: Oral cancer. A practical guide to understanding oral cancer. ELLM Press, 2002

[21] Coussens LM, Fingleton B, Matrisian LM: Matrix metalloproteinase inhibitors and cancer: trials and tribulations. *Science* 295:2387-2392, 2002

[22] Dang CV, Semenza GL: Oncogenic alterations of metabolism. *Trends Biochem. Sci.* 24:68-72, 1999

[23] Dietrich T, Reichart PA, Scheifele C: Clinical risk factors of oral leukoplakia in a representative sample of the US population *Oral Oncol.* 40:158-163, 2004

[24] Dikshit RP, Ramadas K, Hashibe M, Thomas G, Somanathan T, Sankaranarayanan R: Association between diabetes mellitus and pre-malignant oral diseases: a cross sectional study in Kerala, India. *Int. J. Cancer* 118:453-457, 2006

[25] Duffy MJ: The role of proteolytic enzymes in cancer invasion and metastasis. *Clin. Exp. Metast.* 10:145-155, 1992

[26] Gibson J, Lamey PJ, Lewis MAO, Frier BM: Oral manifestations of previously undiagnosed non-insulin dependent diabetes mellitus. *J. Oral Pathol. Med.* 19:284-287, 1990

[27] Gillison ML, Koch WM, Capone RB, Spafford M, Westra WH, LiWu, Zahurak ML, Daniel RW, Viglione MI, Symer DE, Shah KV, Sidransky D: Evidence for a casual association between human papilloma virus and a subset of head and neck cancers. *J. Natl. Cancer Inst.* 92:709-720, 2000.

[28] Golub LM, Lee HM, Greenwald RA, Ryan ME, Sorsa T, Salo T, Glannobile WV: A matrix metalloproteinase inhibitor reduces bone-type collagen degeneration fragments and specific collagenases in gingival crevicular fluid during adult periodontitis. *Inflamm. Res.* 46:310-319, 1997

[29] Gould GW, Holman GD: The glucose transporter family: structure, function and tissue-specific expression. *Biochem. J.* 295:329-341, 1993

[30] Goutzanis L, Vairaktaris E, Yapijakis C, Kavantzas N, Nkenke E, Derka S, Vassiliou S, Acyl Y, Kessler P, Stavrianeas N, Perrea D, Donta I, Skandalakis P, Patsouris E: Diabetes may increase risk for oral cancer through the insulin receptor substrate-1 and focal adhesion kinase pathway. *Oral Oncol.* 43:165-173, 2007

[31] Greenwald RA, Golub LM, Ramamurthy NS, Chowdhury M, Moak SA, Sorsa T: In vitro sensitivity of the three mammalian collagenases to tetracycline inhibition: relationship to bone and cartilage degradation. *Bone* 22:33-38, 1998

[32] Guggenheimer J, Moore PA, Rossie K, Myers D, Mongelluzo MB, Block HM, Weyant R, Orchard T: Insulin-dependent diabetes mellitus and oral soft tissue pathologies. II Prevalence and characteristics of Candida and candidal lesions. *Oral Surg. Oral Med. Oral Pathol. Oral Radiol. Endod.* 89:507-576, 2000.

[33] Hammarsten J, Hogstedt B: Hyperinsulinaemia: A prospectiv risk factor for lethal clinical prostate cancer. *Eur. J. Cancer* 41:2887-2895, 2005

[34] Hashibe M, Jacob BJ, Thomas G: Socioeconomic status, lifestyle factors and oral premalignant lesions. *Oral Oncol.* 39:664-671, 2003

[35] Hu G: Gender difference in all-cause and cardiovascular mortality related to hyperglycaemia and newly-diagnosed diabetes. *Diabetologia* 46:608-617, 2003

[36] Hussain SP, Hofseth LJ, Harris CC: Radical causes of cancer. *Nat. Rev. Cancer* 3:276-285, 2003

[37] Huycke MM, Gaskins HR: Commensal bacteria, redox stress and colorectal cancer: mechanisms and models. *Exp. Biol. Med.* 229:586-597, 2004

[38] Jee SH, Ohrr H, Sull JW, YunJE, Ji M, Samet JM: Fasting serum glucose level and cancer risk in Korean men and women. *JAMA* 293:194-202, 2005

[39] Johnson NW: Etiology and risk factors for oral cancer, with special reference to- bacco and alcohol use. *Hungarian Oncol.* (in Hungarian) 45:115-122, 2001

[40] Jordan RCK, Macabeo-Ong M, Shiboski CH, Dekker N, Ginzinger DG, Wong DTW, Schmidt BL: Overexpression of matrix metalloproteinase-1 and –9mRNA is associated with progression of oral dysplasia to cancer. *Clin. Cancer Res.* 10:6460-6465, 2004

[41] Karin M, Lawrence T, Nizet V: Innate immunity gone awey: linking microbial infections to chronic inflammation and cancer. *Cell* 124:823-835, 2006.

[42] Kinane DF, Chestnutt IG: Smoking and periodontal disease. *Critical Rev. Oral Biol. Med.* 11:356-365, 2000

[43] Kirstein M, Aston C, Hintz R, Vlassara H: Receptor-specific induction of insulin-like growth factor I in human monocytes by advanced glycosylation end product-modified proteins. *J. Clin. Invest*, 90:439-446, 1992

[44] Koistinen HA, Zierath JR: Regulation of glucose transport an human sceletal muscle. *Ann. Med.* 34:410-418, 2003

[45] Krone CA, Ely JTA: Controlling hyperglycemia as an adjunct to cancer therapy. *Integr. Cancer Ther.* 4:25-31, 2005

[46] Kunkel M, Reichert TE, Benz P: Overexpression of Glut-1 and increased metabolism in tumors are associated with poor prognosis in patients with oral squamous cell carcinoma. *Cancer* 97:1015-1024, 2003

[47] Kuriki K, Hirose K, Tajima K: Diabetes and cancer risk for all and specific sites among Japanese men and women. *Eur. J. Cancer Prev.* 16:83-89, 2007

[48] Lax AJ, Thomas W: How bacteria could cause cancer: one step at a time. *Trends Microbiol.* 10:293-299, 2000

[49] Listgarten MA, Ricker FH, Laster L, Shapiro J, CohenDW: Vascular basement membrane lamina thickness in the normal and inflamed gingiva of diabetics and non-diabetics. *J. Periodontol.* 45:676-684, 1974

[50] Manoucher-Pour M, Spagnuolo PJ, Rodman HM, Bissada NF: Comparison of neutrophil chemotactic response in diabetic patients with mild and severe periodontal disease. *J. Periodontol.* 52:410-415, 1981

[51] Mc Mullen JA, Van Dyke TE, Horoszewicz HU, Genco RJ: Neutrophil chemotaxis in individuals with advanced periodontal disease and a genetic predisposition to diabetes mellitus. *J. Periodontol.* 52:167-173, 1981

[52] Mealey BL, Moritz AJ: Hormonal influences: effects of diabetes mellitus and endogenous female sex steroid hormones on the periodontium. *Periodontol* 2000. 32:59-81, 2003

[53] Meyer M, Schreck R, Muller JM, Baeuerle PA: Redox control of gene expression by eukaryotic transcription factors NF-6B, AP-1, and SRF/TCF. In: Pasquier C, Olivier RY, Auclair C, Packer L. (Eds.), Oxidative Stress, Cell Activation and Viral Infection. Birkhauser Verlag, Basel, pp. 217-235, 1994

[54] Meyerhardt JA, Catalano PJ, Haller DG, Mayer RJ, Macdonald JS, Benson AB, Fuchs CS: Impact of diabetes mellitus on outcomes in patients with colon cancer. *J. Clin. Oncol.* 21:433-440, 2003

[55] Mogyorósi A, Ziyadeh FN: GLUT1 and TGF-beta: the link between hyperglycaemia and diabetic nephropathy. *Nephrol. Dial Transplant* 14:2827-2831, 1999

[56] Monnier VM, Glomb M, Elgawish A, Sell DR: The mechanism of collagen cross-linking in diabetes. A puzzle nearing resolution. *Diabetes* 45:67-72, 1996.

[57] Neville BW, Day TA: Tumors and precancerous lesions of the oral cavity. CA *Cancer J. Clin.* 52:195-215, 2002

[58] Nunez NP, Oh WJ, Rozenberg J, Perella C, Anver M, Barrett JC, Perkins SN, Berrigan D, Moitra J, Varticovski L, Hursting SD, Vinson C: Accelerated tumor formation in a fatless mouse with type 2 diabetes and inflammation. *Cancer Res.* 66:5469-5476, 2006

[59] Oliver RJ, Woodwards RT, Sloan P: Prognostic value of facilitative glucose transporter Glut-1 in oral squamous cell carcinomas treated by surgical resection; results of EORTC Transplantational Research Fund studies. *Eur. J. Cancer* 2004; 40: 503-508

[60] Park SM, Lim MK, Shin SA, Yun YH: Impact of prediagnosis smoking, alcohol, obesity, and insulin resistance on survival in male cancer patients: National Health Insurance Corporation Study. *J. Clin. Oncol.* 24:5017-5024, 2006

[61] Philip M, Rowley DA, Schreiber H: Inflammation as a tumor promoter in cancer induction. *Seminars Cancer Biol.* 14:433-439, 2004

[62] Polette M, Clavel C, Muller D et al: Detection of mRNAs encoding collagenase-I and stromelysin-2 in carcinomas of the head and neck by in situ hybridization. *Invasion Metast.* 11:76-83,1991

[63] Rai B, Kharb S, Jain R, Anand, SC: Salivary vitamins E and C in oral cancer. *Redox Report* 12:163-164, 2007

[64] Rapp K, Schroeder J, Klenk J, Ulmer H, Concin H, Diem G, Oberaigner W, Weiland SK: Fasting blood glucose and cancer risk in a cohort of more than 140,000 adults in Austria. *Diabetologia* 49: 945-952, 2006

[65] Reiser KM: Nonenzymatic glycation of collagen in aging and diabetes. *Proc. Soc. Exp. Biol. Med.* 218:23-37, 1998

[66] Ryan M, Ramamurthy NS, Sorsa T, Golub LM: MMP-mediated events in diabetes. *Ann. New York Acad. Sci.* 878: 313-334, 1999

[67] Reichart PA, Philipsen HP: Oral erythroplakia a review. *Oral Oncology* 41:551-561, 2005

[68] Rosenquist K, Wennerberg J, Schildt EB, Bladstrom A, Goran HB, Andersson G: Oral status, oral infections and some lifestyle factors as risk factors for oral and oropharyngeal squamous cell carcinoma. A population-based case-control study in southern Sweden. *Acta Otolaryngol.* 125:1327-1336, 2005

[69] Salahudeen AK, Kanji V, Reckelhoff JF: Pathogenesis of diabetic nephropathy: a radical approach. *Nephrol. Dial Transpl.* 12:664-668, 1997

[70] Sasahira T, Kirita T, Bhawal UK, Yamamoto K, Ohmori H, Fujii K, Kuniyasu H: Receptor for advanced glycation end products (RAGE) is important in the prediction of recurrence in human oral squamous cell carcinoma. *Histopatology* 51:166-172, 2007

[71] Schmidt AM, Hori O, Cao R: RAGE a novel cellular receptor for advanced glycation end products. *Diabetes* 45:77-80, 1996

[72] Schmidt AM, Weidman E, Lalla E, Yan SD, Hori O, Cao R, Brett JG, Lamster IB: Advanced glycation end products (AGEs) induce oxidant stress in the gingiva: a

potential mechanism underlying accelerated periodontal disease associated with diabetes. *J. Periodontal. Res.* 31:508-515, 1996

[73] Soskolne WA: Epidemiological and clinical aspects of periodontal diseases in diabetics. *Ann. Periodontol.* 3:3-12, 1998

[74] Sreebny LM, Yu A, Green A, Valdini A: Xerostomia in diabetes mellitus. *Diabetes Care* 15:900-904, 1992.

[75] Stattin P, Bjor O, Ferrari P, Lukanova A, Lenner P, Lindahl B, Hallmans G, Kaaks R: Prospective study of hyperglycemia and cancer risk. *Diabetes Care* 30:561-567, 2007

[76] Suba Zs, Barabás J, Szabó Gy, Takács D, Ujpál M: Increased prevalence of diabetes and obesity in patients with salivary gland tumors. *Diabetes Care* 28:228, 2005

[77] Suba Zs, Ujpál M: Disorders of glucose metabolism and oral cancer risk. *Fogorv Szle* 100:250-257, 2007

[78] Tezal M, Sullivan MA, Reid ME, Marshall JR, Hyland A, Loree T, Lillis C, Hauck L, Wactawski-Wende J, Scannapieco FA: Chronic periodontitis and the risk of tongue cancer. *Head Neck Surg.* 133:450-454, 2007

[79] Tirosh A, Potashnik R, Bashan N, Rudich A: Oxidative stress disrupts insulin-induced cellular redistribution of insulin receptor sustrate-1 and phosphatidylinositol 3-kinase in 3T3-L1 adipocytes. *J. Biol. Chem.* 274:10595-10602, 1999

[80] Tsuji S, Kawai N, Tsuji M, Kawano S, Hori M. Review article: inflammation-related promotion of gastrointestinal carcinogenesis: a perigenetic pathway. *Aliment Pharmacol. Ther.* 18:82-89, 2003

[81] Ujpál M, Matos O. Bíbok Gy, Somogyi A, Szabó Gy, Suba Zs: Diabetes and oral tumors in Hungary: Epidemiological correlations. *Diabetes Care* 27:770-774, 2004.

[82] Ujpál M, Barabás J, Kovalszky I, Szabó Gy, Németh Zs, Gábris K, Suba Zs: A preliminary comparative study of the prognostic implications of type 2 diabetes mellitus for patients with primary gingival carcinoma treated with surgery and radiation therapy. *J. Oral Maxillofac Surg.* 65:452-456, 2007

[83] Vlassara H, Brownle M, Monogue K, Dinarello CA, Pasagian A: Cachetin/TNF and IL-I induced by glucose-modified proteins: role in normal tissue remodelling. *Science* 240:1546-1548, 1988.

[84] Vlassara H: Recent progress in advanced glycation, end products and diabetic complications. *Diabetes* 46:19-25, 1997

[85] Warburg O: On the origin of cancer cells. *Science* (Wash DC), 123:309-314, 1956

[86] Wild S et al: Global prevalence of diabetes estimates for the year 2000 and projections for 2030. *Diabetes Care* 27:1047-1053, 2004

[87] Yamamoto E, Miyakawa A, Kohama G: Mode of invasion and lymph node metastasis in squamous cell carcinoma of the oral cavity. *Head Neck Surg.* 6:938-947, 1984

[88] Yoshizaki T, Maruyama Y, Sato H, Furukawa M: Expression of tissue inhibitor of matrix metalloproteinase-2 correlates with activation of matrix metalloproteinase-2 and predicts poor prognosis in tongue squamous cell carcinoma. *Int. J. Cancer*, 95:44-50, 2001

Chapter 4

The Role of Estrogen in Health and Disease

Is Estrogen Good Girl or Bad Girl? (Reckelhoff)

For many years, female sexual steroids were considered simply the most important hormones involved in female physiology and reproduction. Nowadays it has become familiar that their actions are much wider than previously thought. Female sexual steroids have crucial roles in many biologic processes [11,16]. Estrogen receptors are fairly involved in gene regulation, cell differentiation and proliferation and have an important role both in male and female physiology. However, our current knowledge probably covers only a small part of their capacities.

Both male and female sexual steroids play an important role in mediating or protecting against cardiovascular diseases and hypertension [47,137]. It is a well-known fact that a physiological estrogen milieu in healthy premenopausal women supplies protection against hypertension and cardiovascular diseases as compared with men of the same age. This has been attributed to the protective effects of estrogens [126]. However, after menopause a rapidly increasing prevalence of ischemic stroke, myocardial infarction and pulmonary emboli among women could be observed.

At the same time, there are many contradictions concerning the associations of female sexual steroids and cancer. Many authors emphasized advantageous impacts of estrogen on metabolic processes [11], gene regulation [16] and longevity [6], whereas others published that estrogen has genotoxic, mutagenic and carcinogenic activities [18,106].

The aim of this chapter is to discuss the fairly contradictory theories concerning the capacities of estrogen based on experimental and clinical investigations.

Biological Effects of Sexual Steroids

In both males and females, the hypothalamus secretes gonadotropin-releasing hormone, which stimulates the anterior pituitary release of both luteinizing and follicular-stimulating hormones. Luteinizing hormone binds to receptors on the ovarian thecal cells in females and on Leydig cells in the testes of males. Follicular-stimulating hormone binds to receptors on ovarian granulosa cells in females or Sertoli cells in males and stimulates the synthesis of aromatase, which converts testosterone to estradiol. A fine-tuned equilibrium of male and female sexual steroids has crucial role in health maintenance.

Both estrogen and androgen receptors are transcriptional factors that bind to the promoter regions of genes. In addition to genomic effects sexual steroids also have nongenomic actions [47,126].

Advantageous Biological Effects of Estrogen

Estradiol has an *antihypertensive effect* through downregulation of some components of the renin-angiotensin system (RAS). Results of animal experiments support that estradiol decreases the expression of angiotensin-1 (AT1) receptors in the kidney vessels [70,121], moreover, it reduces the expression and activity of angiotensin I-converting enzyme [47,56].

Estrogen should be *cardiovascular protective* as it has been shown to inhibit vasoconstrictor activity of endothelin, which is an important regulator of vessel capacities. In healthy premenopausal women, vasodilatator effect of endothelin was predominant [49]. In male-to-female transsexuals estradiol treatment caused a significant reduction in serum endothelin level [160]. In animal experiments estradiol treatment [35] or its metabolites [45] have been shown to inhibit endothelin synthesis and to improve endothelial dysfunction in ovarectomized spontaneously hypertensive rats [166].

Estradiol should also be protective by means of its *antimitogenic effects*. In animal experiments it was protective against neointimal proliferation in female rats [116]. Estradiol and some of its metabolites proved to be antimitogenic in human smooth muscle cells [9], mesangial cells [171] and cardiac fibroblasts [46].

Estradiol has also *antioxidant activities* and protects against oxidative stress [34,163], which has causative role in endothelial dysfunction associated with hypertension [67] and in DNA injuries leading to malignization. In eumenorrhoic women cyclic variation in the antioxidant parameters of the plasma were observed, which could be attributed to cyclic changes in estradiol levels [113]. In clinical studies on essential hypertension, women had lower levels of plasma hydrogen peroxide than did men [93]. Premenopausal women have also been shown to have lower levels of oxidative stress than do men or postmenopausal women [149]. Antioxidant activity of estrogen is protective against atherosclerotic vessel injuries and cancer initiation.

Estradiol decreases the *serum level of bioavailable IGF-I.* Estradiol administration in clinical studies lowered concentrations of total and ultrafiltrably free IGF-I and elevated the level of IGF-I binding protein, which mean a limitation of IGF-I bioavailability. However, testosterone treatment caused elevation of the bioavailable IGF-1 level [162]. Elevated level of free IGF-I is characteristic of hyperinsulinemia and insulin resistance, which are well-known etiologic factors for both cardiovascular diseases and malignancies [17]. Estrogen induced lower bioavailability of IGF-1 seems to be equivocally advantageous against these severe diseases.

Nowadays, estrogen and its receptors have been shown to be advantageous regulators of *glucose homeostasis*, insulin sensitivity and cellular glucose uptake by modulation of the expression of several genes [11]. Recently, glucose metabolism disorders have been regarded as crucial risk factors for both cardiovascular diseases and cancer [17]. These correlations support that estrogen induced increase in insulin sensitivity is an important protective factor. Associations of estrogen and insulin signals are discussed in details in the Chapter 7.

Estrogens have also beneficial impact on serum lipid level, lipid composition and *lipid metabolism* [164], which affects advantageously the insulin sensitivity. As dyslipidemia is a strong risk factor for both cardiovascular diseases and cancers, regulation of the lipid composition in the serum and the different tissues by estrogen means an antiatherogenic and anticancer capacity.

Anti-inflammatory effects of estradiol are well known based on both clinical and experimental studies [6,137]. There are gender related differences in the inflammatory response and survival following hemorrhage and subsequent sepsis [42,172]. The inhibitory action of estrogen in the process of inflammation may rely on the prevention of chemokines to recruit effector immune cells [59]. Estrogen suppresses lung inflammatory reactions in mice through an effect on vascular cell adhesion molecules and proinflammatory mediator substances [146].

There are studies on the anti-inflammatory actions of both types of estrogen receptors (ERs). ERβ. In vitro experiments revealed a blocking effect of estradiol on the induction of CD40 and CD40L expression and prevention of neutrophil adhesion by means of a pathway mediated by Erα [61]. ER-β selective agonists in several animal models of human diseases showed also an unexpected anti-inflammatory impact [69]. In vitro studies suggested that anti-inflammatory effects of ER-β selective estrogens may be attributed to transcriptional reproduction of proinflammatory genes [33].

These inhibitory effects on inflammatory reactions should be advantageous against intimal lesions and atheromatous plaque formation in the arterial walls [148]. Moreover, quenching effect of estrogen on chronic inflammations is a segment of its anticancer capacity as long lasting inflammatory processes are proven predecessors of malignancies at several sites [152,155].

Estradiol increases the *activity of the immunologic system*. However, high immune reactivity among females creates a delusive favor. Though it is advantageous against infectious diseases, and even malignancies, it is detrimental in terms of increased development of allergic and autoimmune diseases [92].

Cytokines interfere with steroidgenesis at the level of adrenals, testes and ovaries [20]. In undifferentiated ovarian cells TNF-alpha and IL-1 inhibit the synthesis of steroid hormones, whereas in differentiated ovaries inflammatory cytokines may stimulate it. As cytokines and corticosteroid hormones have mainly antagonistic roles in the immunologic processes their regulation is a great power in the immunologic reactivity. Increased immunoreactivity may also have an important role in anticancer capacity.

Anticancer effect of estrogen has been justified in animal experiments. Testosterone treatment or ovarectomy increased the incidence of carcinogen induced renal cell carcinoma in female rats, whereas estradiol treatment or castration decreased the tumor incidence in male animals [37]. An endogenous metabolite of estradiol (2-methoxyestradiol) showed antitumor effects on human melanoma cell lines as well as in male mice after intrasplenic injection of human melanoma cells [43].

Cardiovascular Complications in Premenopausal Women with Type-2 Diabetes and in Postmenopausal Cases

Failures of beneficial antiatherogenic effect of estrogen were reported in premenopausal women with type-2 diabetes, and in postmenopausal cases.

Premenopausal women with type-2 diabetes had a greater incidence of aortic stiffening [36] and left ventricular hypertrophy [25] and similar or higher risk for cardiovascular mortality as compared with men [77,86].

It is not clear why premenopausal, hormonally active women are not protected from vascular complications of diabetes. However, studies to evaluate serum estradiol levels in premenopausal diabetic women, especially those who do not have strict glycemic control, have not been performed [137]. A plausible explanation of the high incidence of cardiovascular events among premenopausal women with type-2 diabetes may be the compromised biosynthesis of estradiol in chronic metabolic diseases.

In postmenopausal women, failure of estrogen therapy to defend atherosclerotic processes is not rare [137]. In these cases unsuccessful treatment may be attributed to the earlier developed definite vascular lesions. It is possible that earlier starting of hormone therapy during perimenopause, before onset of vascular injuries, may prove more beneficial against cardiovascular diseases.

In postmenopausal cases, increase in blood pressure does not occur at once as a woman passes menopause but after at least a 5-year interval [26]. This suggests that though loss of estrogen may be the primary mediator of postmenopausal hypertension, other age-related secondary factors, such as insulin resistance may have a role in the risk for cardiovascular diseases.

Epidemiological studies supported that coronary disease showed the same or even poorer outcome in postmenopausal women as compared with men, though in most of the studies women were considerably older than men [62,119]. In postmenopausal cases decreased estrogen level is in close association with decreased insulin sensitivity [169] and this double harmful effect may be the clue to the increased vulnerability of the cardiovascular system. Close correlations of estrogen deficiency and insulin resistance will be discussed in the Chapter 7.

Androgens, Cardiovascular Diseases and Cancer Risk

Androgen hormones have some quite opposite effects as compared with estrogens causing hypertension, anabolic, cell proliferating activity, inhibition of apoptosis and stimulation of oxidative stress [137]. These data justify that the risk for cardiovascular diseases, hypertension and cancer may be higher among middle-aged men as compared with women.

Men have higher blood pressure than women throughout most of their lives, and cardiovascular disease (CVD) develops at an earlier age in men than in women [26]. Results of animal experiments support that CVD may be mediated by androgens in males [54,127] but the exact mechanisms by which androgens may mediate CVD and hypertension have not been clarified.

Recently testosterone was reported to be able to induce a direct *stimulation of sodium resorption* through the proximal tubules of the kidney [133]. Androgen receptors were localized to the proximal tubules [90], and androgens could affect the synthesis of the RAS components [29]. These effects of androgens may influence blood pressure by means of different mechanisms.

Vasoconstrictor production is a further mechanism by which androgens may provoke CVD and hypertension. Renin activity in the plasma is regularly higher in men than in premenopausal women [85]. Castration decreases and testosterone treatment increases the expression of messenger RNA for angiotensinogen and renin in kidneys of hypertensive rats [29]. Female to male transsexuals receiving testosterone treatment have an elevated serum endothelin level as compared with untreated females [160]. Thus, androgens may cause increased blood pressure and endothelial dysfunction by means of increased vasoconstriction.

Male sexual steroids may *stimulate oxidative stress*, which promotes the development of CVD and hypertension [136]. Androgens increase superoxide production, which could quench the bioactivity of nitric oxide and may cause vasoconstriction by several routes. Increased oxidative stress caused by androgens may play a pivotal role in cardiovascular risk in men. Nevertheless, excessive free radical deliberation may have a role in cancer risk in man especially for tumors showing very high male to female ratio.

Young sportsmen treated with anabolic steroids show *insulin resistance* and its early cardiovascular complications [32]. Low or high doses of androgen treatment resulted in increased blood pressure both in young and older men [63]. Excessive androgen production and estrogen deficiency in women is associated with increased prevalence of metabolic syndrome and type-2 diabetes [120], which are risk factors for both cardiovascular events and cancer.

Female Longevity and its Sources

Female longevity is an evergreen subject of both medicine and biology. Historically women live longer than men almost all over the world. Everybody knows the differences between the two sexes in the development and manifestations of cardiovascular disease. However, for all main causes of death, including heart disease, cerebrovascular lesions, cancer, chronic pulmonary diseases and accidents males die at a higher rate as compared with women [6].

In a review study, several hypotheses were analyzed, which were proposed for gender differences in longevity [6]. One hypothesis is that estrogen hormone at cellular level somehow protects females and this is the clue to their longer life. A second hypothesis is that females live longer because of their more active immune system [4]. According to the third hypothesis the heterogametic sex is in association with gender related longevity. As males have a single copy of genes they can express the X genes only from their single X chromosome. However, females could have an advantage by selecting the better X chromosome while inactivating the deleterious one. The fourth hypothesis supposes that reduction of the activity of growth hormone and IGF-I signaling cascade result in smaller body and longer life span [23]. The 5th hypothesis attributes the longer life to a decreased oxidative stress. Defense mechanisms against oxidative damages are stronger in women [34,163], which favorably influence both aging and a wide variety of diseases.

The majority of factors presumed to be advantageous for longevity are in close correlation with estrogen and ER signaling. Estrogen mediates advantageous immune reactions following trauma and hemorrhage [4,172]. Moreover, estrogens have pivotal roles in the favorable up-regulation of genes of the antioxidant enzymes, and that of the participants of insulin sensitivity, such as IGF-I [19,34,132,149,162,163]. Moreover, estrogens play important positive role in regulating the growth hormone-IGF-I axis as attenuate the growth hormone action by suppressing growth hormone receptors [99]. Furthermore, normal ovarian female steroid hormone synthesis is associated with two, functioning X-chromosomes [141].

Considering the theories and the results of investigations concerning female longevity, the most important factors affecting the longer life of females may be the gender specific ones. Both the double X chromosomes and the excess of female sexual steroid hormones against androgenic ones are unique, physiologic features in women and these may have decisive role in female longevity. Carcinogenic capacity of estrogen would be a disadvantage for life span of females both among animals and humans.

Hormonal Influences on Longevity and Cancer Risk

The endocrine system may be a key determinant in the evolutionarily well-conserved mechanisms of life span [23]. The endocrine system is highly integrated in mammals and regulates metabolism, growth, reproduction and response to stress among other functions. Changes in one part of the system causing longer or shorter life certainly result in secondary endocrine effects on other functions.

Growth hormone, insulin-like growth factor-I and insulin seem to be at the forefront of hormonal control of aging and disease.

Growth hormone (GH) is a pituitary derived hormone that has functions both in somatic development and metabolic processes. Ames and Snell dwarf mutant mice with GH, prolactin and thyreotropin deficiency exhibit significant extension in life span but small body size and defective fertility [24]. GH deficiency in dwarf mice delayed aging and extended the life span via enhanced antioxidative defense, enhanced stress resistance, increased insulin sensitivity and reduced tumor prevalence [12,15,135].

On the contrary, GH transgenic mice with high GH levels live half as long as wild type siblings [147]. Diabetogenic effect and increased oxidative stress caused by excessive GH production may strongly shorten the life span [7]. In GH transgenic mice high levels of GH and IGF-1 are also associated with accelerated aging and tumor promotion [27].

Insulin and IGF-I have great impact on the level of oxidative stress. Chronic hyperglycemia and hyperinsulinism in insulin resistance are known pro-oxidant factors [112]. Studies have also shown that insulin mediated glucose uptake may be improved by vitamin E administration along with lower plasma free radical concentrations [128]. Metabolic and carcinogenic effects of elevated insulin and IGF levels are discussed in Chapter 2.

Thyroid hormones may also play important but fairly controversial role in longevity and cancer initiation. Thyroid hormones are prime regulators of intermediary metabolism in virtually every tissue, and their action is mediated by binding and activation of the nuclear receptors [154]. They can up-regulate enzymes and cytochromes involved in mitochondrial function [167].

Thyroid hormones have important role in longevity regulation [125]. In thyroid hormone deficient, dwarf mice the reduced metabolism and decreased oxidative damage may contribute to their longer life span [139].

Longevity studies on very old patients (>85) revealed that decreased levels of free thyroxin were strongly associated with longer life span [66,130]. A plausible explanation for these data may be that necessity for thyroid hormones may gradually decrease during the life span. In young adults higher physical and mental activity, reproductive capacity and anabolic processes require accelerated fuel oxidation and higher rate of metabolism. Low thyroid hormone levels in elderly patients may be the characteristics of the aging process, which cannot justify that lifelong hypothyroidism would be advantageous.

A study on middle-aged males with subclinical hypothyroidism showed a higher rate of mortality from all causes [83]. Hypothyroidism also shows close associations with dyslipidemia, insulin resistance and cardiovascular diseases [159]. Recently, our working group revealed significant correlation between hypothyroidism and oral cancer risk among non smoker, non drinker women. Possible correlations between hypothyroidism and cancer risk will be discussed in the Chapter 8.

Sexual steroid hormones have a finical equilibrium both in males and females. In males androgens, in females estrogens exhibit a great predominance. Though overproduction or deficiency of near all hormones cause characteristic diseases, in case of sexual steroids mainly their relation may be altered [23]. These disorders may cause feminization in males and virilization in females.

Pathological overproduction of estrogen hormone is extremely rare, such as in case of tumors with hormone production. However, recent results revealed that asymptomatic, lifelong, moderate estrogen deficiency is relatively frequent in women and may have an onset in young girls. Its pathologic base is generally the polycystic ovary [142]. These estrogen deficiency states affect not only the fertility, but may also cause serious metabolic and gene regulation disorders leading to increased risk for cardiovascular diseases.

Changes in sexual steroid equilibrium are closely associated with alterations in insulin sensitivity [120]. Excess of androgens and the concomitant estrogen deficiency are in close correlation with insulin resistance in both genders, though the ideal ratio of the male and female sexual steroids is fairly different in men and women. Associations of insulin resistance, estrogen deficiency and cancer will be discussed in the Chapter 7.

Summary of Associations among Hormones, Longevity and Cancer Risk

Considering the associations between the endocrine system and longevity it may be established that health and longevity require a stable equilibrium and harmony among the hormonal signals. Complexity of the endocrine system determines that both high and low levels of any hormone result in further changes in the whole hormonal system and lead to severe diseases. Like in an orchestra, in the endocrine system one dissonant instrument will completely spoil the concordance of the whole performance.

The associations between hormonal disorders and cancer risk are much more controversial. Overproduction of peptide hormones such as growth hormone, insulin and IGFs, which trigger biochemical signals upon interacting with their cell membrane receptors, have proven tumor-inducing capacity.

Another group of hormones including estrogens and thyroids have genomic, intranuclear and non-genomic receptor signals, thus both of them initiate transcriptional activity by several pathways. Estrogen deficiency emerged as cancer risk factor for oral cancer cases [150]. In a recent Hungarian study thyroid hormone deficiency also showed close correlations with oral cancer risk among non smoker, non drinker women (Chapter 8).

Literary Data Supporting the Carcinogenic Capacity of Estrogen

Nowadays, a prevailing concept is the positive correlation between female sexual steroid hormones and risk for cancers at several sites [38,50,53,78,106]. Theoretically, the assumption concerning carcinogenicity of excessive estrogen would be plausible but fortunately, the ER signal pathways are strictly protected because of their pivotal importance [16]. Nevertheless, review of the literary data concerning the carcinogenic capacity of estrogen reveals more and more confusion and contradiction in this field.

Assumed Carcinogenic Capacity of Estrogen Based on Animal Experiments

Tumor induction capacity of natural estrogen was first reported based on animal experiments in the early 1940s [107]. Since that time more reports on tumor induction by estrogen on rodent models have been published [91,122,165].

In these animal models, tumors were developed using high, pharmacological estrogen doses with the aim to examine the carcinogenic activity of the hormone in a relatively short period of time. Increased cancer incidence was observed at several sites both in highly and moderately estrogen dependent organs, as ERs are widespread all over the body of mammals.

In mice, high estrogen level increased the incidence of mammary, pituitary, endometrial, cervical, vaginal, testicular, lymphoid and bone tumors [75,81,117]. In rats, estrogen administration increased the incidence of mammary and pituitary tumors [84,122,143]. In hamsters, a high incidence of malignant kidney tumors occurred in intact and castrated males after estrogen administration [91,100,103].

However, there were no animal models in which physiological doses of estrogen could induce tumors. Nevertheless, predicting value of carcinogenicity testing at such high doses of estrogen has been fairly questionable [1].

Epidemiological Data Suggesting Carcinogenic Capacity of Estrogen in Humans

Potential carcinogenic activity of estrogen in humans had not been published for many years till the early 1980s. This long lasting silence concerning the carcinogenic effect of estrogen in humans may be explained by the fact that diseases with excessive estrogen production are extremely rare. This may explain that possible carcinogenic capacity of estrogen was of no interest to human medicine.

Widespread use of contraceptives and hormone replacement therapy among postmenopausal women brought a breakthrough at the end of the last century. From the early 1980s epidemiological and clinical studies have increasingly pointed to an elevated breast, endometrial and ovarian cancer risk associated with estrogens [13,14,31,38,52,60,88,97,144].

Even a slightly elevated serum level of endogenous estrogen was regarded as risk for breast cancer [13,52,89,153]. However, other clinical studies failed to identify any association between elevated serum hormone levels and breast cancer [60,170].

Exogenous estrogens alone or in combination with progestin were found to be also risk factors for breast cancer [31,74,79,88,131] summarized the results of population based epidemiological studies that had been published supporting the relative breast cancer risk from use of hormone replacement therapy. However, from the 10 studies reviewed only 5 showed statistically significant positive association between hormone treatment and breast cancer risk, whereas the other 5 could not justify this. Moreover, in the Women's Health Initiative randomised trial on postmenopausal women with hysterectomy estrogen treatment was associated with a possible reduction in breast cancer risk [3]

Although no randomised, controlled double blind studies have been conducted, the available literary data suggested that use of estrogen replacement therapy for more than 5-10 years means an increased relative risk for breast cancer [106].

Many epidemiologists accepted exogenous estrogen administration as a risk factor for human endometrial carcinoma [64,108,144]. An increased risk was established with increasing doses of estrogen and with the length of treatment [88]. However, an increased risk for endometrial cancer in association with HRT has not been justified either by the Women's Health Initiative (WHI) randomised trial [2] or by the Heart and Estrogen/Progestin Replacement Study (HERS) [80].

Carcinogenic activity of steroidal estrogens has been summarized by the IARC, which classified the evidences for these effects in humans [82].

Assumptions for the Mechanism of Estrogen Carcinogenicity

There is a widespread agreement among scientists that carcinogenesis in hormone sensitive tissues is not possible without a contribution by receptor-mediated hormonal effects [106]. Recently, it has become well known that estradiol and its receptors regulate in conjunction with other hormones and mediators the development, differentiation and later the proper function and metabolism of all organs [11,16]. Discriminative separation of some "hormone sensitive" organs from other hormone responsive organs regarding differences in their carcinogenic processes is fairly questionable.

The principle of *hormonal contribution of estrogen to carcinogenesis* is based on its physiologic functions in gene regulation by means of nuclear and plasma membrane receptors [40]. In vitro inhibition of estrogen-induced proliferation of human tumor cell line by hormone antagonists was evaluated as a crucial role of estrogen receptors in hormone dependent tumor growth [87]. In Syrian hamsters renal carcinogenesis induced by excessive estrogen doses was also inhibited by hormone antagonists [105]. An alternatively proposed carcinogenic mechanism was the binding of estrogen to a regulatory plasma protein and cancelling its inhibitory effect on cell proliferation [145]. All these data suggested that estrogen-regulated proliferation of highly hormone sensitive cells might fix spontaneous or induced DNA damage and thus establish a potentially malignant tumor [106].

A series of bacterial and mammalian gene mutation assays failed to justify any *mutagenic activity of estrogens* [101,118]. For instance, estrogens do not display any mutagenic activity in the Ames (Salmonella typhimurium) assay with or without an extrinsic metabolising system [95]. Estrogens also failed to induce mutations in V79 Chinese hamster cells when tested in high concentrations [44,134]. Moreover, estradiol did not induce sister chromatid exchanges in human lymphocytes, whereas the synthetic diethylstilbestrol did generate such alterations [76].

This failure of justifying mutagenic capacity of estrogen led several researchers to propose various epigenetic pathways of tumor induction.

Epigenetic, estrogen-induced carcinogenesis by uncontrolled stimulation of mammary epithelial cell proliferation was proposed in the early 80s [55]. A modification of this proposal was the ER-mediated proliferation of mammary epithelial cells carrying spontaneous replication errors [52]. However, the absence of ERs in proliferating human mammary epithelial cells [30,140] provided evidence against this proposed carcinogenic pathway.

A receptor-mediated stimulation of growth factors by estrogen in neighbouring cells emerged as indirect stimulation of mammary epithelial cell proliferation [40]. However, synthetic estrogens with well-maintained hormonal potency showed fairly low carcinogenicity in animal models [104]. These latter results indicated that errors of spontaneous replication of normal cells may not be sufficient for tumor development solely in response to proliferative stimuli.

Carcinogenesis by covalent modification of estrogen receptors was also a proposed mechanism [21]. This hypothesis assumed that an estradiol metabolite, the 16α-hydroxyestrone covalently binds to the amino groups of estrogen receptor protein. Through this route the metabolite permanently stimulates the receptor and induces gene expression and cell proliferation in an uncontrolled manner [151]. Covalent binding of estrogens including catecholestrogen metabolites to DNA was first reported by Liehr and co-workers [5]. However, other scientists could not justify the mechanism of estrogen-induced carcinogenesis by covalent modification of estrogen receptors [158].

Estrogen induced chromosomal abnormalities emerged also as plausible explanation of carcinogenicity. However, estrogen induced neoplastic transformation of Syrian hamster embryo cells was reported without detectable concomitant gene mutations [10,156]. Neither synthetic nor natural estrogens caused detectable gene mutations, whereas concomitant aneuploidity occurred with cell transformation [157]. Syrian hamster embryo cells with spontaneous chromosomal mutations were not capable to induce tumors in nude mice [48]. These results suggested that in addition to spontaneous chromosomal abnormalities other genetic changes (mutations) are necessary for cells to acquire carcinogenic capacity.

Li and co-workers proposed an *epigenotoxic, multistage scheme* for estrogen induced carcinogenesis in the hamster kidney [102] as they detected only very low rates of metabolic conversion of estradiol to catechol metabolites. Epigenotoxic carcinogen was defined as an agent that is not involved in direct (covalent) or indirect interactions with the genetic material but is able to elicit heritable changes by alternative mechanisms. This new hypothesis was also based on the failure to confirm the formation of estrogen induced DNA adducts [39].

However, Li and associates questioned the ability of estrogens and their metabolites to induce DNA damage in the carcinogenesis process [101]. They found insufficient concentration of estradiol in the target tissues for hormone-induced cancer and the rate of its conversion to catecholestrogen was too low to result in significant amounts of genotoxic metabolites.

This critique was based upon the measurement of low plasma estrogen levels. However, the ratio of mammary tissue to plasma estrogen levels approximates 1:1 in premenopausal women, whereas in postmenopausal cases this ratio may be elevated as high as 10-50:1 [161]. Local concentrations of estrogen in mammary tissue and breast tumor were regarded to depend more likely on the aromatase activity of the mammary cells than on the ovarian hormone supply [114]. In situ aromatase activity was found to be associated with both breast tumor estradiol levels and rate of cellular proliferation [173].

Differences in the ratio of breast tissue: serum estrogen concentrations in pre-menopausal and postmenopausal women raise striking questions. A plausible assumption would be that decreased ovarian hormone production after menopause induces local aromatase activity in the breast tissue to compensate the low serum estrogen level. Like in case of short-circuit, the missing electricity may be substituted by a current-generator so as to save the indispensable functions. In this safety mechanism for maintenance of breast tissue health, estrogen level may rather be defensive than offensive to promote of cancer initiation.

Free radical mediated DNA damage also emerged as an indirect mechanism of estrogen-induced carcinogenesis. DNA single-strand breaks were induced in MCF-7 human breast cancer cells in culture by 3,4-estrone quinone [123]. Similar DNA damage was also induced in vivo in the kidney of Syrian hamsters treated with either estradiol or 4-hydroxyestradiol many months before tumor development [68]. Concentrations of 8-hydroxyguanine DNA bases, formed by hydroxy radical reaction, were increased in DNA incubated with catecholestrogens [115].

However, continuously increasing number of literary data has established that estrogens have definite antioxidant activity and protective effect against oxidative stress especially in premenopausal women [113,137,163]. These protective estrogen effects were discussed earlier.

Estrogen-induced *chromosomal aberrations* affecting growth controlling genes and resulting in tumor development were also reported. Numerical chromosomal changes or genome mutations might be induced by estradiol and other estrogens in cell cultures [157] and in laboratory animals [8]. Both synthetic and natural estrogens also induced structural chromosomal aberrations in addition to numerical changes. Treatment of Syrian hamsters with estradiol resulted in variable structural aberrations such as deletions, inversions and translocations in kidney cells long before tumor development.

However, these types of estrogen-induced chromosomal aberrations may not be sufficient by themselves for tumor development [48]. They may probably contribute to carcinogenesis by compromising the integrity of the genetic material [98].

Controversial Associations of Hormone Replacement Therapy and Cancer Risk

Hormone replacement therapy (HRT) in postmenopausal women has been fairly widespread in the economically developed countries in the past two decades. These cases supply excellent possibilities to study the associations between female sexual steroid hormones and tumor incidence. Till now, the prevailing concept is that HRT is associated with an increased prevalence of gynecological cancers [38,53,97].

However, recent clinical studies on HRT use in postmenopausal women yielded unexpected and fairly controversial associations with malignancies [51,65]. Unexplained, beneficial anticancer effects of HRT use were reported against oral, esophageal, gastric, colorectal, cervical, liver and lung cancers [53,57,97,124,129,138] and there are also contradictory results concerning the associations of HRT and highly hormone dependent cancers [2,3,41]. Controversial associations of endocrine disturbances to cancer development in the hormone dependent organs are discussed in Chapter 6.

Most of the controversies concerning the correlations between estrogen effect and tumors may be found on smoking associated cancers, which exhibit well-known gender-related differences, such as unexplained excess in male cases.

Urinary bladder cancer is a typically smoking associated tumor and its risk is three to four times as great in men than in women [71]. The gender specific high incidence rate of bladder cancer persisted even in the absence of exposure to cigarettes, occupational hazards, or urinary tract infections.

Striking contradictions have been published concerning the associations between HRT and urinary bladder cancer. Among HRT user women an excess risk was found for bladder cancer in a case-control study [53] Other authors could not justify any association of hormone related factors with bladder cancer incidence in women [28]. However, in a follow up study, estrogen deficiency such as postmenopausal status and young age at menopause did unfavorably affect the risk for bladder cancer in women [110]. Similarly, late menopause and longer duration of fertile life correlated with a reduced risk for gastric cancer [96]. In our Hungarian case control study late menopause showed a negative, whereas menopausal state a positive association with oral cancer risk in women [150].

Just as urinary bladder cancer, upper aerodigestive tract tumors are strongly smoking associated too, and their incidence also shows a high male to female ratio. Cancer incidence at these sites exhibits controversial associations with HRT use as well. Laryngeal cancer is the neoplasm with the largest male to female sex ratio in most populations. In a case-control study on women with laryngeal cancer, menstrual and hormonal factors did not appear to have a consistent role in laryngeal carcinogenesis [58].

However, prospective clinical studies justified a protective role of long term HRT (48 months) against smoking associated tumors, such as oral, laryngeal and pharyngeal cancers among current smokers, but did not affect the tumor incidence among non-smokers [124]. The authors supposed that HRT rather postpones than prevents the smoking associated cancers by a transitory maintenance of epithelial thickness and integrity in the upper aero-digestive tract, which may counteract exogenous carcinogenic agents. Unfortunately, the age of the patients and the length of their postmenopausal period were not analyzed in this study. Considering the results of our Hungarian studies on oral cancer cases hormonal effects of HRT use may both prevent and postpone the risk for oral cancer (see Chapter 5).

Lung cancer is also highly smoking-associated tumor and its incidence exhibits high male to female ratio. Studies on correlations between HRT and lung cancer risk in women have reported controversial associations. Recently, HRT use in postmenopausal women was found to be associated with reduced risk for lung cancer independent of smoking status, however, this association was strongest among never smokers [138].

HRT has also anticancer capacities at other tumor sites out of the upper aero-digestive tract such as in stomach, colon, liver and cervix [53,96,129], which can hardly be explained by a local defense mechanism against tobacco products and exogenous carcinogenic agents. HRT probably exerts this advantageous effect by means of its systemic metabolic and hormonal pathways.

Dietel and coworkers revised the current concept of tumor growth dynamics and its controversial associations with HRT [41]. It seemed to be rather questionable whether female hormones may induce malignancies de novo even in hormone sensitive tissues. There was a much more likely assumption that hormones may merely promote the proliferation of already existing, hormone sensitive tumors. The long developmental process of tumors from cancer initiation is also an apparent contradiction to an increased cancer risk in HRT users within a 1-5 years period. Critique of the correlations between HRT use and cancer risk is discussed in Chapter 6.

Revision of Results Concerning Carcinogenic Capacity of Estrogen

In case of estrogen, which has complex roles in gene regulation affecting cell growth, proliferation and differentiation, use of excessive hormone doses may evidently cause many disturbances. All experimental results, which successfully supported the carcinogenic capacity of estrogen, were assessed under fairly unnatural circumstances. These experimental data justified that estrogen is a great power of Nature but in wrong hands it becomes a risky weapon.

In experimental animals excessive overdosage of estrogen could initiate tumors in several organs disregarding their hormone sensitivity, however, these results were not consequently equivocal and reproducible. Moreover, rodents included into these studies are short-lived and with aging an increased prevalence of spontaneous tumors may also be deceiving.

In vitro experiments trying to clarify the carcinogenic mechanism of estrogen effect, were fairly simplified models disregarding the cross talks and feed back mechanisms of mediators under biological circumstances. Nevertheless, all failures to justify the carcinogenic capacity of estrogen were evaluated as a result of shortcomings of the methods employed. Finally, estrogen proved to be a "weak" carcinogen based on the controversial experimental results concerning its mutagenic and genotoxic activity.

In humans even physiological levels of endogenous or therapeutic estrogens have been regarded as carcinogenic agents but preferentially for the highly estrogen sensitive organs. Cancers may be induced either by weak or strong carcinogens depending on the inherited inclination, presence of other risk factors, as well as further circumstances. However, widespread HRT use justified an inverse, anticancer effect of estrogen at several sites, even in highly hormone sensitive organs, which cannot be reconciled with the carcinogenic capacity of estrogen.

Summarizing the literary data concerning the carcinogenic capacity of estrogen, there are many contradictions and shortcomings both in the experimental and clinical results. Failures in forced justification of the carcinogenic effects of estrogen served as proofs for high safety of its gene regulatory mechanisms.

Physiologically Elevated Level of Female Sexual Steroids in Humans

A common physiological state is pregnancy when the serum levels of female sexual steroids, growth hormones and growth factors are highly elevated. Nevertheless, till now there are no literary data suggesting that pregnancy and delivery mean an increased cancer risk either in the highly or moderately estrogen sensitive organs. In contrast, literary data support the protective effect of parity and breast-feeding against breast cancer [22].

It is a well-known fact that in case of abortion the highly elevated estrogen level is followed by an abrupt decrease. However, there are fairly controversial data concerning the correlations between abortion, miscarriage and breast cancer incidence [168].

Some authors reported on a declining breast cancer risk as the number of induced abortions increased [109] Further epidemiological evidences were presented that induced abortions do not affect women's risk of having breast cancer [111]. Other authors established an increased breast cancer risk in connection with abortions [94], especially in cases of long gestation period [72]. Among women with late terminations, such as fifth months or later, there were twice as many breast cancers as expected. As late abortion and abrupt decrease of highly elevated estrogen level is a drastic shock to the breast tissue, the latter results seem to be well established.

Female sexual steroids have a unique role in commanding the abrupt tissue proliferation processes both in the female genital tract during pregnancy and in all tissues of embryonic development. Estrogen receptors (ERα and ERβ) are widely distributed in different tissues, with the predominance of one or the other isoform [16]. In murine mammary epithelial cell lines selective agonists for ERα caused dominantly cell proliferation whereas agonists for ERβ inhibited the cell growth and mitotic activity [73]. Equilibrium of the activity of estrogen receptors may be a crucial moderator of growth, development, differentiation and metabolism in all tissues. Carcinogenic potential of estrogen in physiological doses would be a failure of Nature.

References

[1] Ames BN, Shigenaga MK, Gold LS: DNA lesions, inducible DNA repair, and cell division: three key factors in mutagenesis and carcinogenesis. *Environ Health Perspect* 101:35-44, 1993

[2] Anderos GL, Judd HL, Kaunitz AM, et al: Women's Health Initiative Investigator Effects of estrogen plus progestin on gynaecologic cancers and associated diagnostic procedures: The Women's Health Initative randomised trial. *JAMA* 290:1739-1748, 2003

[3] Anderson GL, Limacher M, Assaf AR, Bassford T, Beresford SA, Black H, Bonds D, Brunner R, Brzyski R, Caan B, Chlebowski R, Curb D, Gass M, Hays J, Heiss G, Hendrix S, Howard BV, Hsia J, Hubbell A, Jackson R, Johnson KC, Judd H, Kotchen JM, Kuller L, LaCroix AZ, Lane D, Langer RD, Lasser N, Lewis CE, Manson J, Margolis K, Ockene J, O'Sullian MJ, Phillips L, Prentice RL, Ritenbaugh C, Robbins J, Rossouw JE, Sarto G, Stefanick ML, Van Horn L, Wactawski-Wende J, Wallace R, Wassertheil-Smoller S: Women's Health Intitative Steering Committee. Effects of conjugated equine estrogen in postmenopausal women with hysterctomy: the Women's Health Intitative randomized controlled trial. *JAMA* 291:1701-1712, 2004

[4] Angele MK, Schwacha MG, Ayala A,Chaudry IH: Effect of gender and sex hormones on immune responses following shock. *Shock*, 14:81-90, 2000

[5] Ashburn SP, Han X, Liehr JG: Microsomal hydroxylation of 2-and 4-fluorestradiol to catechol metabolites and their conversion to methyl ethers: catechol estrogens as possible mediators of hormonal carcinogenesis. *Mol. Pharmacol.* 43:534-541, 1993

[6] Austad SN: Why women live longer than men: Sex differences in longevity. *Gender Medicine* 3:79-92, 2006

[7] Balbits A, Bartke A, Turyn D: Overexpression of bovine growth hormone in transgenic mice is associated with changes in hepatic insulin receptors and their kinase activity. *Life Sci.* 59:1362-1371, 1996

[8] Banerjee SK, Banerjee S, Li SA, Li JJ: Induction of chromosome aberrations in Syrian hamster renal cortical cells by various estrogens. *Mutat. Res.* 311:191-197, 1994

[9] Barchiesi F, Jackson E, Gillespie D, Zacharia L, Fingerle J, Dudey RK: Methoxyestradiols mediate estradiol-induced antimitogenesis in human aortic SMCs. *Hypertension* 39: 874-879, 2002

[10] Barrett JC, Wong A, McLachlan JA: Diethylstilbestrol induces neoplastic transformation without measurable gene mutation at two loci. *Science* 212:1402-1404, 1981

[11] Barros RPA, Machado UF, Gustafsson JA: Estrogen receptors: new players in diabetes mellitus. *Trends in Molecular Medicine* 9: 425-431, 2006

[12] Bartke A, Brown-Borg HM: Life extension in the dwarf mouse. *Curr. Top. Dev. Biol.* 63:189-225, 2004

[13] Bernstein L: The epidemiology of breast cancer. *LOWAC J.* 1:7-13, 1998

[14] Berrino F, Muti P, Micheli A, Bolelli G, Krogh V, Sciajno R, Pisani P, Panico S, Secreto G: Serum sex hormone levels after menopause and subsequent breast cancer. *J. Natl. Cancer Inst.* 88:291-296, 1996

[15] Bielschowsky F, Bielschowsky M: Carcinogenesis in the pituitary of dwarf mouse. The response to dimethylbenzanthracene applied to the skin. Br J Cancer 15:257-262, 1961

[16] Björnström L, Sjöberg M: Mechanisms of estrogen receptor signaling: Convergence of genomic and nongenomic actions on target genes. *Molecular Endocrinol.* 19:833-842, 2005

[17] Bloomgarden ZT: Definitions of the insulin resistace syndrome: The 1st Word Congress on the Insulin Resistance Syndrome. *Diabetes Care* 27:824, 2004

[18] Bolton JL, Thatcher GR: Potential mechanisms of estrogen quinone carcinogenesis. *Chem. Res. Toxicol.* 21:93-101, 2008

[19] Borras C, Sastre J, Garcia-Sala D et al: Mitochondria from females exhibit higher antioxidant gene expression and lower oxidative damage than males. *Free Radic. Biol. Med.* 34:546-552, 2003

[20] Bornstein SR, Rutkowski H, Vrezas I: Cytokines and steroidgenesis. *Molecular and Cell Endocrin.* 215:135-141, 2004

[21] Bradlow HL, Hershcopf RJ, Martucci CP, Fishman J: Estradiol 16α-hydroxylation in the mouse correlates with mammary tumor incidence and presence of murine mammary tumor virus: a possible model for the hormonal etiology of breast cancer in humans. *Proc. Natl. Acad. Sci. USA* 82:6295-6299, 1985

[22] Britt K, Ashworth A, Smalley M: Pregnancy and the risk of breast cancer. *Endocrine-Related Cancer* 14:907-933, 2007

[23] Brown-Borg HM: Endocrine regulation of longevity. *Ageing Research Reviews* 6:28-45, 2007

[24] Brown-Borg HM, Borg KE, Meliska CJ, Bartke A: Dwarf mice and the ageing process. *Nature* 384:33, 1996

[25] Bruno G, Giunti S, Bargero G, Ferrero S, Pagano G, Perin P: Sex-differences in prevalence of electrocardiographic left ventricular hypertrophy in type 2 diabetes: the Casale Monferrato Study. *Diabetes Med.* 21:823-828, 2004

[26] Burl VL, Whelton P, Roccella EJ, Brown C, Cutler JA, Higgins M, Horan MJ, Labarthe D: Prevalence of Hypertension in the US Adult Population. Results From the Third National Health and Nutrition Examination Survey, 1988-1991. *Hypertension* 25:305-313, 1995

[27] Burroughs KD, Dunn SE, Barrett JC, Taylor JA: Insulin-like growth factor-I: a key regulator of human cancer risk? *J. Natl. Cancer Inst.* 91:579-581, 1999

[28] Cantwell MM, Lacey JV Jr, Schairer C, Schatzkin A, Michaud DS: Reproductive factors, exogenous hormone use and bladder cancer risk in a prospective study. *Internatiolnal Journal of Cancer* 119:2398-2401, 2006

[29] Chen Y-F, Naftilan AJ, Oparil S: Androgen-Dependent Angiotensinogen and Renin Messenger RNA Expression in Hypertensive Rats. *Hypertension* 19:456-463, 1992

[30] Clark RB, Howell A, Potten CS, Anderson E: Dissociation between steroid receptor expression and cell proliferation in human breast. *Cancer Res.* 57:4987-4991, 1997

[31] Colditz GA, Hankinson SE, Hunter DJ, Willett WC, Manson JE, Stampfer MJ, Hennekens C, Rosner B, Speizer FE: The use of estrogens and progestins and the risk of breast cancer in postmenopausal women. *N Engl. J. Med.* 332:1589-1593, 1995

[32] Cohen JC, Hickman R: Insulin resistance and diminished glucose tolerance in powerlifters ingesting anabolic steroids. *J. Clin. Endocrinol. Metab.* 64:960-963, 1987

[33] Cvoro A, Tatomer D, Tee MK, Zogovic T, Harris HA, Leitman DC: Selective estrogen receptor-beta agonists repress transcription of proinflammatory genes. *J. Immunol.* 180:630-636, 2008

[34] Dantas A, Tostes R, Fortes A, Costa S, Nigro D, Carvalho M: In vivo evidence for antioxidant potential of estrogen in microvessels of female spontaneously hypertensive rats. *Hypertension* 39:405-411, 2002

[35] David FL, Carvalho MH, Cobra AL, Nigro D, Fortes ZB, Reboucas NA, Tostes RC: Ovarian hormones modulate endothelin-1 vascular reactivity and mRNA expression in DOCA-salt hypertensive rats. *Hypertension* 38:692-696, 2001

[36] DeAngelis I, Millasseau S, Smith A, Viberti G, Jones R, Ritter J, Chowienczyk P: Sex differences in age-related stiffening of the aorta in subjects with type 2 diabetes. *Hypertension* 44:67-71, 2004

[37] Deguchi J, Miyamoto M, Okada S: Sex hormone-dependent renal cell carcinogenesis induced by ferric nitrilotriacetate in Wistar rats. Jpn J Cancer Res 86: 1068-1071, 1995

[38] Diamanti-Kandarakis E: Hormone replacement therapy and risk of malignancy. *Curr. Opinion Obstet Gynecol.* 16:73-78, 2004

[39] DiAugustine RP, Walker M, Li SA, Li JJ: DNA adduct profiles in hamster kidney following chronic exposureto various carcinogenic and non-carcinogenic estrogens. In: Li JJ, Nandi S, Li SA (eds) Hormonal Carcinogenesis. Springer-Verlag, New York, pp 293-297, 1992

[40] Dickson RB, Gelmann EP, Knabbe C, Jasid K, Bates S, Swain S: Mechanisms of estrogenic and antiestrogenic regulation of growth of human breast carcinoma. In: Klijn JGM, (ed) Hormonal Manipulation of Cancer: Peptides, Growth Factors, and New (Anti) Steroidal Agents. Raven Press, New York, pp381-403, 1987

[41] Dietel M, Lewis MA, Shapiro S: Hormone replacement therapy: pathobiological aspects of hormone-sensitive cancers in women relevant to epidemiological studies on HRT: a mini-review. *Human Reproduction* 20:2052-2060, 2005

[42] Diodato MD, Knöferi MW, Schwacha MG,Bland KI,Chaudry IH: Gender differences in the inflammatory response and survival following hemorrhage and subsequent sepsis. *Cytokine,* 14:162-169, 2001

[43] Dobos J, Tímár J, Bocsi J, Burian Zs, Nagy K, Barna G, Petak I, Ladányi A: In vitro and in vivo antitumor effect of 2-methoxyestradiol on human melanoma. *Int. J. Cancer* 112:771-776, 2004

[44] Drevon C, Piccoli C, Montesano R: Mutagenity assays of estrogenic hormones in mammalian cells. *Mutat. Res.* 89:83-90, 1981

[45] Dubey RK, Jackwson E, Keller P, Imthurm B, Rosselli M: Estradiol metabolites inhibit endothelin synthesis by an estrogen receptor-independent mechanism. *Hypertension* 37:640-644, 2001

[46] Dubey R, Gillespie D, Zacharia L, Rposselli M, Imthurn B, Jackson E. Methoxyestradiols mediate the antimitogenic effects of locally applied estradiol on cardiac fibroblast growth. *Hypertension* 39:412-417, 2002

[47] Dubey RK, Oparil S, Imthurn B, Jackson EK: Sex hormones and hypertension. *Cardiovasc Res.* 53:688-708, 2002

[48] Endo S, Metzler M, Hieber L: Nonrandom karyotypic changes in a spontaneously immortalized and tumorigenic Syrian hamster embryo cell line. *Carcinogenesis* 15:2387-2390, 1994

[49] Ergul A, Shoemaker K, Puett D, Tackett RL: Gender differences in the expression of endothelin receptors in human saphenous veins in vitro. *J. Pharmacol. Exp. Ther.* 285 .511-517, 1998

[50] ESHRE Capri Workshop Group: Hormones and breast cancer. *Human Reprod. Update* 10:281-293, 2004

[51] Ettinger B, Friedman GD, Bush T, Quesenberry CP Jr: Reduced mortality associated with long-term postmenopausal estrogen therapy. *Obstet Gynecol.* 87: 6-12, 1996

[52] Feigelson HS, Henderson BE: Estrogens and breast cancer. *Carcinogenesis* 17:2279-2284, 1996

[53] Fernandez E, Gallus S, Bosetti C, Franceschi S, Negri E, La Vecchia C: Hormone replacement therapy and cancer risk: a systematic analysis from a network of case-control studies. *Int. J. Cancer* 105:408-412, 2003

[54] Fortepiani LA, Yanes LL, Zhang H, Racusen LC, Reckelhoff JF: Role of androgens in mediating renal injury in aging SHR. *Hypertension* 42:952-955, 2003

[55] Furth J: Hormones as etiological agents in neoplasia. In: Becker FF (ed) Cancer. A Comprehensive Treatise.1. Etiology: Chemical and Physical Carcinogenesis. Plenum Press, New York, Chapt 4:89-134, 1982

[56] Gallagher P, Li P, Lenhart J, Chappel M, Brosnihan K: Estrogen regulation of antiogestin-converting enzyme mRNA. *Hypertension* 33:323-328, 1999

[57] Gallus S, Bosetti C, Franceschi S, Levi F, Simonato L, Negri E, La Vecchia C: Oesophageal cancer in women: tobacco, alcohol, nutritional and hormonal factors. *Br. J. Cancer* 85:341-345, 2001

[58] Gallus S, Bosetti C, Franceschi S, Levi F, Negri E, LaVecchia C: Laryngeal cancer in women. Tobacco, alcohol, nutritional, and hormonal factors. *Cancer Epidemiol. Biomark Prev.* 12:512-517, 2003

[59] Garidou L, Laffont S, Douin-Echinard V, Coureau C, Krust A, Chambon P, Guery JC: Estrogen receptor (alpha) signaling in inflammatory leukocytes is dispensable for

17(beta)-estradiol-mediated inhibition of experimental autoimmune encephalomyelitis. *J. Immunol.* 173:2436-2442, 2004

[60] Garland CF, Friedlander NJ, Barrett-Conner E, Khaw KT: Sex hormones and postmenopausal breast cancer: a prospective study in an adult community. *Am. J. Epidemiol.* 135:1220-1230, 1992

[61] Geraldes P, Gagnon S, Hadjadj S, Merhi Y, Sirois MG, Cloutier I, Tanguay JF: Estradiol blocks the induction of CD40 and CD40L expression on endothelial cells and prevents neutrophil adhesion: an ER-alpha-mediated pathway. *Cardiovasc. Res.* 71: 566-573, 2006

[62] Gottlieb S, Harpaz D, Shotan A, Boyko V, Leor J, Cohen M, Mandelzweig B, Mazouz B, Stern S, Behar S: Sex differences in management and outdome after acute myocardial infarction in the 1990's: A prospective observational community-based study. Israel Thrombolytic Survey Group. *Circulation* 102:2484-2490, 2000

[63] Grace F, Sculthorpe N, Baker J, Davies B: Blood pressure and rate pressure product response in males using high-dose anabolic androgenic steroids. (AAS). *J. Sci. Med. Sport* 6:307-312, 2003

[64] Greenwald P, Caputo TA, Wolfgang PE: Endometrial cancer after menopausal use of estrogens. *Obstet Gynecol.* 50:239-243, 1977

[65] Grodstein F, Clarkson T, Manson J: Understanding the divergent data on postmenopausal hormone therapy. *N Engl. J. Med.* 348: 645-650, 2003

[66] Gussekloo J, van Exel E, de Craen AJ,Meinders AE, Frolich M, Westendorp RG: Thyroid status, disability and cognitive function and survival in old age. *JAMA* 292:2591-2599

[67] Hamilton C, Brosnan M, McIntyre M, Graham D, Dominiczak A. Superoxide excess in hypertension and aging: A common cause of endothelial dysfunction. *Hypertension* 37:529-534, 2001

[68] Han X, Liehr JG: DNA single strand breaks in kidneys of Syrian hamsters treated with steroidal estrogens. Hormone induced free radical damage preceding renal malignancy. *Carcinogenesis* 15:977-1000, 1994

[69] Harris HA, Albert LM, Leathurby Y et al: Evaluation of an estrogen receptor-beta agonist in animal models of human disease. *Endocrinology* 147:2085-2085, 2006

[70] Harrison-Bernard L, Schulman I, Raij L: Postovariectomy hypertension is linked to increased renal AT1 receptor and salt sensitivity. *Hypertension* 42:1157-1163, 2003

[71] Hartge P, Harvey EB, Linehan WJ, Silverman DT, Sullivan JW, Hoover RN, Fraumeni JF: Unexplained Excess Risk of Bladder Cancer in Men. *J. Natl. Cancer Inst.* 82:1636-1640, 1990

[72] Hartge P: Abortion, breast cancer and epidemiology. N Engl J Med 336:127-128, 1997

[73] Helguero LA et al: Estrogen receptors α (ERα) and β (ERβ) differentially regulate proliferation and apoptosis of the normal murine mammary epithelial cell line HC11. *Oncogene* 24:6605-6616, 2005

[74] Henderson BE, Ross RK, Pike MC: Hormonal chemoprevention of cancer in women. *Science* 259:633-638, 1993

[75] Highman B, Greenman DL, Norvell MJ, Farmer J, Shellenberger TE: Neoplastic and preneoplastic lesions induced in female C3H mice by diets containing diethylstilbestrol or 17β-estradiol. *J. Environ. Pathol. Toxicol.* 4:81-95, 1980

[76] Hill A, Wolff S, Sister chromatid exchanges and cell division delays induced by diethylstilbestrol, estradiol and estriol in himan lymphocytes. *Cancer Res.* 43:4114-4118, 1983

[77] Hu G: Gender difference in all-cause and cardiovascular mortality related to hyperglycaemia and newly-diagnosed diabetes. *Diabetologia* 46:608-617, 2003

[78] Huber JC, Schneeberger C, Tempfer CB: Genetic modelling of the estrogen metabolism as risk factor of hormone-dependent disorders. *Maturitas* 20:1-12, 2002

[79] Hulka BS, Liu ET, Lininger RA: Steroid hormones and risk of breast cancer. *Cancer* 74:1111-1124, 1993

[80] Hulley S, Grady D, Busch T, et al: Randomised trial of estrogen plus progestin for secondary prevention of coronary heart disease in postmenopausal women: heart and Estrogen/Progestin Replacement Study (HERS) Research Group. *JAMA* 380:605-613, 1998

[81] Huseby RA: Demonstration of a direct carcinogenic effect of estradiol on Leydig cells of the mouse. *Cancer Res*. 40:1006-1013, 1980

[82] International Agency for Research on Cancer: Monographs on the evaluation of carcinogenic risks to humans: hormonal contraception an postmenopausal hormone therapy. IARC, Lyon, France, vol 72, 1999

[83] Imaizumi M, Akahoshi M, Ichimaru S, Nakashima E, Hida A, Soda M, Usa T, Ashizawa K, Yokoyama N, Maedea R, Nagataki S, Eguchi K: Risk for ischemic heart disease and all-cause mortality in subclinical hypothyroidism. *J. Clin. Endocrinol. Metab*. 89:3365-3370, 2004

[84] Inoh A, Kamiya K, Fujii Y, Yokoro K: Protective effects of progesterone and tamoxifen in estrogen-induced mammary carcinogenesis in ovariectomized W/Fu rats. *Jpn. J. Cancer Res.* 76:699-704, 1985

[85] James GD, Sealey JE, Muller F, Adlerman M Madhavan S, Laragh JH: Renin relationship to sex, race and age in normotensive population. *J. Hypertens.* 4:S387-S389, 1986

[86] Kanaya A, Grady D, Barrett-Connor E: Explaining the sex difference in coronary heart disease mortality among patients with type 2 diabetes mellitus: a meta-analysis. *Arch Intern. Med.* 162:1737-1745, 2002

[87] Katzenellenbogen BS: Estrogen receptors: bioactivity and interactions with cell signaling pathways. *Biol. Reprod.* 54:287-293, 1996

[88] Key TJA, Pike MC: The dose-effect relationship between „unopposed"estrogens and endometrial mitotic rate: its central role in explaining and predicting endometrial cancer risk. *Br. J. Cancer* 57:205-212, 1988

[89] Key TJ, Applyby PN, Reeves GK: Body mass index, serum sex hormones and breast cancer risk in postmenopausal women. *J. Natl. Cancer Inst.* 95: 1218-1226, 2003

[90] Kimura N, Mizokami A, Oonuma T, Sasano H, Nagura H. Immunocytochemical localization of androgen receptor with polyclonal antibody in paraffin-embedded human tissues. *J. Histochem. Cytochem*. 41:671-678, 1993

[91] Kirkman H: Estrogen-induced tumors of the kidney. III. Growth characteristics in the Syrian hamster. *J. Natl. Cancer Inst. Monogr.* 1:1-57, 1959

[92] Klein SL: Hormonal and immunological mechanism mediating sex differences in parasite infection. *Parasite Immunol.* 26:247-264, 2004

[93] Lacy F, O'Connor D, Schmid-Schonbein G: Plasma hydrogenperoxide in hypertensive and normotensive subjects at genetic risk of hypertension. *J. Hypertens.* 16:291-303, 1998

[94] Lanfranchi A: The science study and sociology of the abortion breast cancer link. *Law and Medicine* 21:95-108, 2005

[95] Lang R, Reiman R: Studies for a genotoxic potential of some endogenous and exogenous sex steroids. I. Communication: examination for the induction of gene mutations using the Ames Salmonella/ microsome test and the HGPRT test in V79 cells. *Environ. Mol. Mutagen.* 21:272-304, 1993

[96] La Vecchia C, D'Avanzo B, Franceschi S, Negri E, Parazzini F, Decarli A: Menstrual and reproductive factors and gastric-cancer risk in women. *Int. J. Cancer* 59:761-764, 1994

[97] La Vecchia C, Brinton LA, McTiernan A: Menopause, hormone replacement therapy and cancer. *Maturitas* 39: 97-115, 2001

[98] Lengauer C, Kinzler KW, Vogelstein B: Genetic instabilites in human cancers. *Nature* 396:643-649, 1998

[99] Leung K-Ch, Johansson G, Leong GM, Ho KKY: Estrogen regulation of growth hormone action. *Endocrine Rev.* 25:693-721, 2004

[100] Li JJ, Li SA: Estrogen-induced tumorigenesis in hamsters: roles for hormonal and carcinogenic activities. *Arch Toxicol.* 55:110-118, 1984

[101] Li JJ, Li SA: Estrogen carcinogenesis in hamster tissues: a critical review. *Endocr. Rev.* 11:524-531, 1990

[102] Li JJ, Li SA: Estrogen carcinogenesis in the hamster kidney: a hormone-driven multi-step process. In: Huff J, Boyd J, Barrett JC (eds) Cellular and Molecular Mechanisms of Hormonal Carcinogenesis: Environmental Influences. Wiley-Liss, Philadelphia, pp 255-267, 1996

[103] Liehr JG, Fang WF, Sirbasku DA, Ari-Ulubelen A: Carcinogenicty of catechol estrogens in Syrian hamsters. *J. Steroid. Biochem.* 24:353-356, 1986

[104] Liehr JG, Stancel GM, Chorich LP, Bousfield GR, Ulubelen AA: Hormonal carcinogenesis separation of estrogenicity from carcinogenicity. *Chem. Biol. Interact.* 59:173-184, 1986

[105] Liehr JG, Sirbasku DA, Jurka E, Randerath K, Randerath E: Inhibition of estrogen-induced renal carcinogenesis in male Syrian hamsters by Tamoxifen without decrease in DNA adduct levels. *Cancer Res.* 48:779-783, 1988

[106] Liehr JG: Is estradiol a genotoxic and mutagenic carcinogen? *Endocrine Rev.* 21:40-54, 2000

[107] Lipschutz A, Vargas Jr L, Structure and origin of uterine and extragenital fibroids induced experimentally in the guinea pig by prolonged administration of estrogens. *Cancer Res.* 1:236-248, 1941

[108] MacMahon B: Risk factors for endometrial cancer. *Gynecol. Oncol.* 2:122-129,1974

[109] Mahue-Giangreco M, Ursin G, Sullivan-Halley J, Bernstein L: Induced abortion, miscarriage and breast cancer risk of young women. *Cancer Epidemiol. Biomark and Prev.* 12:209-214, 2003

[110] McGrath M, Michaud DS, De Vivo I: Hormonal and reproductive factors and the risk of bladder cancer in women. *Am. J. Epidemiol.* 163: 236-244, 2006

[111] Melbye M, Wohlfahrt J, Olsen JH et al: Induced abortion and the risk of breast cancer. *N Engl. J. Med.* 336:81-85, 1997

[112] Mezzetti A, Lapenna D, Romano F, Costantini F, Pierdomenico SD, De Cesare D, CuccurulloF, Riario-Sfroza G, Zuliani G, Fellin R: Systemic oxidative stress and its relationship with age and illness. Associazione Medica „Sabin" *J. Am. Geriatr. Soc.* 44:823-827, 1996

[113] Michos C, Kiortsis DN,Evangelou A, Karkabounas S: Antioxidant protection during menstrual cycle: the effects estradiol on ascorbic-dehydroascorbic acid plasma levels and total antioxidant plasma status in eumenorrhoic women during menstrual cycle. *Acta Obstet. Gynecol. Scand.* 85:960-965, 2006

[114] Miller WR, O'Neill J: The importance of local synthesis of estrogen within the brest. *Steroids* 50:537-548, 1987

[115] Mobley JA, Bhat AS, Brueggemeier RW: Measurement of oxidative DNA damage by catechol estogens and analogues in vitro. *Chem. Res. Toxicol.* 12:270-277, 1999

[116] Mori T, Durand J, Chen Y, Thompson J, Bakir S, Oparil S: Effects of short term estrogen treatment on the neointimal response to balloon injury of rat carotid artery. *Am. J. Cardiol.* 85:1276-1279, 2000

[117] Nagasawa H, Mori T, Nakajima Y: Long-term effects of progesterone or diethylstilbestrol with or without estrogen after maturity on mammary tumorigenesis in mice. *Eur. J. Cancer* 16:1583-1589, 1980

[118] Nandi S: Role of hormones in mammary neoplasia. *Cancer Res.* 38:4046-4049, 1978

[119] Natarajan S, Liao Y, Cao G, Lipsitz S, McGee D: Sex differences in risk for coronary heart disease mortality associated with diabetes and established coronary heart disease. *Arch Int. Med.* 163:1735-1740, 2003

[120] Nestler JE: Obesity, insulin, sex steroids and ovulation. *Int. J. of Obesity and Related Metabolic. Disorders* 24: 571-573, 2000

[121] Nickenig G, Baumer AT, Grohe C, Kahlert S, Strehlow K, Rosenkranz S, Stablein A, Beckers F, Smits JFM, Daemen MJAP, Vetter H, Bohm M: Estrogen Modulates AT1 Receptor Gene Expression in Vitro and in Vivo. *Circulation* 97:2197-2201, 1998

[122] Noble RL, Hochacka BC, King D: Spontaneous and estrogen-produced tumors in Nb rats and behaviour after transplantation. *Cancer Res.* 35:766-780, 1975

[123] Nutter LM, Ngo EO, Abul-Hajj YY: Characterization of DNA damage induced by 3,4-estrone-o-quinone in human cells. *J. Biol. Chem.* 226:16380-16386, 1991

[124] Olsson H, Bladström AM, Ingvar C: Are smoking-associated cancers prevented or postponed in women using hormone replacement therapy? *Obstet Gynecol.* 102: 565-570, 2003

[125] Ooka H, Shinkai T: Effects of hyperthyreoidism on the life span of the rat. *Mech. Age Dev.* 33:275-282, 1986

[126] Orshal JM, Khalil RA: Gender, sex hormones and vascular tone. *Am. J. Physiol. Regul. Integ. Comp. Physiol.* 286:R233-R249, 2004

[127] Ouchi Y, Share L, Crofton JT, Iitake K, Brooks DP: Sex Difference in the Development of Deoxycorticosterone-Salt Hypertension in the Rat. *Hypertension* 9:172-177, 1987

[128] Paolisso G, Tagliamonte MR, Rizzo MR, Manzella D, Gambardella A, Varricho M: Oxidative stress and advancing age: results in healthy centenarians. *J. Am. Geriatr. Soc.* 46:833-838, 1998

[129] Parazzini F, La Vecchia C, Negri E, Franceschi S, Bolis G: Case-control study of estrogen replacement therapy and risk of cervical cancer. *Br. Med. J.* 315: 85-88, 1997

[130] Parle JV, Maisonneuve P, Sheppard MC, Boyle P, Franklyn JA: Prediction of all-cause and cardiovascular mortality in elderly people from one low serum thyrotropin results: a 10-year cohort study. *Lancet* 358:861-865, 2001

[131] Pike M, Bernstein L, Spicer D: Exogenous hormones and breast cancer risk. In: *Neiderhuber J,* (ed) Current Therapy in Oncol BC Decker, St. Louis, MO, pp 292-302, 1993

[132] Prottegente AR, England TG, Rehman A et al: Gender differences in steady-state levels of oxidative damage to DNA in healthy individuals. *Free Radic. Res.* 36:157-162, 2002

[133] Quan A, Chakravarty S, Chen J-K, Chen J-C, Loleh S, Saini N, Harris R, Capdevila J, Quigley R: Androgens augment proximal tubule transport. *Am. J. Physiol. Renal. Physiol.* 287.452-459, 2004

[134] Rajah TT, Pento JT: The mutagenic potential of antiestrogens at the HPRT locus in V79 cells. Res. *Commun. Mol. Pathol. Pharmacol.* 89:85-92, 1995

[135] Ramsey MM, Ingram RL, Cashion AB, Ng AH, Cline JM, Parlow AF, Sonntag WE: Growth hormone-defitient dwarf animals are resistant to dimethylbenzantracine (DMBA)-induced mammary carcinogenesis. *Endocrinology* 143:4139-4142, 2002

[136] Reckelhoff J, Romero J: Role of oxidative stress in angiotensin-induced hypertension. *Am. J. Physiol. Regul. Integr. Comp. Physiol.* 284:893-912, 2003

[137] Reckelhoff JF: Sex steroids, cardiovascular disease, and hypertension. *Hypertension* 45: 170-174, 2005

[138] Rodriguez C, Feigelson HS, Deka A, Patel AV, Jacobs EJ, Thun MJ, Calle EE: Postmenopausal hormone therapy and lung cancer risk in the Cancer Prevention Study II Nutrition Cohort. *Cancer Epidemiol. Biomark and Prev.* 17:655-660, 2008

[139] Romanick Ma, Rakoczy SG,Brown-Borg HM: Long-lived Ames dwarf mouse exhibits increased antioxydant defense in skeletal muscle. *Mech. Ageing Dev.* 125:269-281, 2004

[140] Russo J, Ao X, Grill C, Russo IH: Pattern of dirtibution of cells positive for estrogen receptor α and progesterone receptor in relation to proliferating cells in the mammary gland. *Breast Cancer Res. Treat* 53:217-227, 1999

[141] Santoro N: Mechanisms of premature ovarian failure. *Ann. Endocrinol.* (Paris) 64:87-92, 2003

[142] Sartor BM, Dickey R: Polycystic ovarian syndrome and the metabolic syndrome. *Am. J. Med. Sci.* 330:336-342,2005

[143] Shull JD, Spady TJ, Snyder MC, Johansson SL, Pennington KL: Ovary intact, but not ovariectomized female ACI rats treated with 17β-estradiol rapidly develop mammary carcinoma. *Carcinogenesis* 18:1595-1601, 1997

[144] Siiteri PK, Nisker JA, Hammond GL: Hormonal basis of risk factors for breast and endometrial cancer. In: Iacobelli S, King RJB, Lindner HR, Lippman ME. (eds) *Hormones and Cancer.* Raven Press, New York, pp 499-505, 1980

[145] Soto AM, Sonnenschein C: Regulation of cell proliferation: is the ultimate control positive or negative? In: Iversen OH (ed) New Frontiers in Cancer Causation. Proceedings of the Second International Conference on Theories of Carcinogenesis. Taylor and Francis, Washington, DC, Chap 9:109-123, 1993

[146] Speyer CL, Rancilio NJ, McClintock ShD, Crawford JD, Gao H, Sarma JV, Ward PA: Regulatory effects of estrogen on acute lung inflammation in mice. *Am. J. Physiol. Cell Physiol.* 288: C881-C890, 2005

[147] Steger RW, Bartke A, Cecim M: Premature aging in transgenic mice expressing growth hormone genes. *J. Repro. Fertil.* 46:61-75, 1993

[148] Stork S, von Schacky C, Angerer P: The effect of 17-estradiol on endothelial and inflammatory markers in postmenopausal women: a randomized, controlled trial. *Atherosclerosis* 165:301-307, 2002

[149] Strehlow K, Rotter S, Wassmann S, Adam O, Grohe C, Laufs K, Bohm M, Nickenig G. Modulation of antioxidant enzyme expression and function by estrogen. *Circ. Res.* 93:170-177, 2003.

[150] Suba Zs: Gender-related hormonal risk factors for oral cancer. *Pathol Oncol. Res.* 13:195-202, 2007

[151] Swaneck GE, Fishman J: Covalent binding of the endogenous estrogen 16α-hydroxyestrone to estradiol receptor in human breast cancer cells: characterization and intranuclear localization. *Proc. Natl. Acad. Sci. USA* 85:7831-7835, 1988

[152] Tezal M, Sullivan MA, Reid ME, Marshall JR, Hyland A, Loree T, Lillis C, Hauck L, Wactawski-Wende J, Scannapieco FA: Chronic periodontitis and the risk of tongue cancer. *Head and Neck Surg.* 133:450-454, 2007

[153] Toniolo PG, Levitz M, Zeleniuch-Jacquotte A, Banerjee S, Koenig KL, Shore RE, Strax P, Pasternack BS: A prospective study of endogenous estrogens and breast cancer in post-menopausal women. *J. Natl. Cancer Inst.* 86:1076-1082, 1995

[154] Tsai MJ, O'Malley BW: Molecular mechanisms of action of steroid / thyroid receptor superfamily members. *Annu. Rev. Biochem.* 63:451-486, 1994

[155] Tsuji S, Kawai N, Tsuji M, Kawano S, Hori M. Review article: inflammation-related promotion of gastrointestinal carcinogenesis: a perigenetic pathway. *Aliment Pharmacol. Ther.* 18:82-89, 2003

[156] Tsutsui T, Suzuki N, Fukuda S, Sato M, Maisumi H, McLachlan JA, Barrett JC: 17β-Estradiol-induced cell transformation and aneuploidy of Syrian hamster embryo cells in culture. *Carcinogenesis* 8:1715-1719, 1987

[157] Tsutsui T, Barrett JC: Neoplastic transformation of cultured mammalian cells by estrogens and estrogen-like chemicals. *Environ. Health Perspect* 105 supp 3:619-624, 1997

[158] Ursin G, London S, Stanczyk FZ, Gentzschein E, Paganini Hill A, Ross RK, Pike MC: Urinary 2-hydroxyestrone/16α-hydroxyestrone ratio and risk of breast cancer in postmenopausal women. *J. Natl. Cancer Inst.* 91:1067-1072, 1999

[159] Uzunlulu M, Yorulmaz E, Oguz A: Prevalence of subclinical hypothyroidism in patients with metabolic syndrome. *Endocrine J.* 54:71-76, 2007

[160] Van Kesteren PJ, Kooistra T, Lansink M, van Kamp GJ, Asscheman H, Gooren LJ, Emeis JJ, Vischer UM, Stehouwer CD: The effects of sex steroids on plasma levels of marker proteins of endothelial cell functioning. *Thromb Haemost* 79:1029-1033, 1998

[161] Van Landeghem AAJ, Poortman J, Nabuurs M, Thijssen JH: Endogenous concentration and subcellular distribution of estrogens in normal and malignant breast tissue. *Cancer Res.* 45:2900-2906, 1985

[162] Veldhuis JD, Frystyk J, Iranmanesh A, Orskov H: Testosterone and estradiol regulate free insulin-like growth factor I (IGF-I), IGF binding protein (IGFBP-I), and dimeric IGF-I/IGFBP-I concentrations. *J. Clin Endocrin. and Metab.* 90:2941-2947, 2005

[163] Vina J, Sastre J, Pallardo FV, Gambini J, Borras C: Role of mitochondrial oxidative stress to explain the different longevity between genders. Protective effect of estrogens. *Free Radic. Res.* 40:1359-1365, 2006

[164] Walsh BW, Schiff I, Rosner B, Greenberg L, Ravinkar V, Sacks FM: Effect of postmenopausal estrogen replacement on the concentrations and metabolism of plasma lipoproteins. *N Engl. J. Med.* 326:954-955, 1992

[165] Welsch CW, Adams C, Lambrecht LK, Hassett CC, Brooks CL: 17β-Oestradiol and Enovid mammary tumorigenesis in C3H/HeJ female mice: counteraction by concurrent 2-bromo-α-ergocryptine. *Br. J. Cancer* 35:322-328, 1977

[166] Widder J, Pelzer T, VonPoser-Klein C, Hu K, Jazbutyte F, Fritzemeier K-H, Hegele-Hartung C, Neyses L, Bauersachs J: Improvement of endothelial dysfunction by selective estrogen receptor-alpha stimulation of ovariectomized SHR. *Hypertension* 42:991-996, 2003

[167] Wiesner RJ, Kurowski TT, Zak R: Regulation by thyroid hormone of nuclear and mitochondrial genes encoding subunits of cytochrome-c oxidase in rat liver and skeletal muscle. *Mol. Endocrinol.* 6:1458-1467, 1992

[168] Wingo PA, Newsome K, Marks JS, Calle EE, Parker SL: The risk of breast cancer following spontaneous or induced abortion. *Cancer Causes Control* 8:260, 1997

[169] Wu ShI, Chou P, Tsai ShT: The impact of years since menopause on the development of impaired glucose tolerance. *J. Clin. Epidemiol.* 54:117-120, 2001

[170] Wysowski KK, Comstock GW, Helsing KJ, Lau HL: Sex hormone levels in serum in relation to the development of breast cancer. *Am. J. Epidemiol.* 125:791-799, 1987

[171] Xiao S, Gillespie D, Baylis C, Jackson E, Dudey R. Effects of estradiol and its metabolites on glomerular endothelial nitric oxide synthesis and mesangial cell growth. *Hypertension* 37:645-650, 2001

[172] Yokoyama Y, Schwacha MG, Samy TS, Bland KI, Chaudry IH: Gender dimorphism in immune responses following trauma and hemorrhage. *Immunol. Res.* 26:63-76, 2002

[173] Yue W, Wang JP, Hamilton CJ, Demers LM, Santen RJ: In situ aromatization enhances breast tumor estradiol levels and cellular proliferation. *Cancer Res.* 58:927-932, 1998

Chapter 5

Estrogen Deficiency as Cancer Risk Factor

A Heretical Idea

The majority of cancers at different sites have a fairly large male to female sex ratio. Moreover, the mean age of female cases with cancer is conspicuously higher as compared with males. These gender-related differences are especially striking concerning the so-called highly smoking associated malignancies such as cancers of the upper aerodigestive tract and the urinary bladder [27].

Oral cancer is a typically smoking-related cancer with fairly high male to female incidence ratio (see Chapter 1). Besides the conspicuously lower incidence of women among oral cancer patients, female cases are significantly older as compared with males. For a long time, the high prevalence of male cases among oral cancer patients had been attributed to the excessive smoking and alcohol consumption and to their synergistic carcinogenic effect. However, the differences in the smoking habits and alcohol consumption between the tumor-free male and female populations are not high enough to justify this concept. Further, the accumulation of oral cancer cases among non smoker, non drinker elderly females remained a further mystery to be answered.

The gender specific risk for oral cancer suggests some endocrine involvement in the epidemiology of this tumor and raises two different assumptions. First, there might be noxious factors affecting predominantly the male patients. Second, though common risk factors affect both sexes, women have some defense mechanisms in their generative period owing to special hormonal and metabolic features.

Though oral cancer is a multicausal disease, till now the exogenous harmful noxae (tobacco, excessive alcohol intake and dietary factors) were overemphasized in its epidemiology (see Chapter 1). Recently, the decreasing frequency of tobacco use and alcohol intake in many populations could not effectively eradicate the occurrence of oral cancer and the gender related differences remained conspicuous among oral cancer cases.

Our working group was the first in clearing up that a systemic disorder; type-2 diabetes is also a strong risk factor for both oral precancerous lesions and cancers. These results were obtained on pooled male-female populations of oral cancer patients and tumor-free controls. Since than, further studies followed, which strengthened this correlation between type-2 diabetes and oral cancer risk (see Chapter 3).

Gender Related Risk Factors for Oral Cancer: Estrogen Deficiency and Elevated Fasting Glucose (Hungarian Case-Control Study)

The aim of the presented case-control study was to examine the role of some systemic risk factors in oral cancer epidemiology separately on male and female cases and to answer the following questions:

1. What is the explanation for the conspicuous excess of male oral cancer cases?
2. Why are the female cases significantly older than males among oral cancer cases?
3. Is there any correlation between the reproductive factors of women and their oral cancer risk?
4. Could there be any gender related association between elevated fasting glucose level and oral cancer risk?

A total of 2660 inpatients (530 females and 2130 males) at the Department of Oral and Maxillofacial Surgery with histologically confirmed squamous cell oral carcinoma (OC) were included in a case-control study between 1 January 1997 and 30 June 2006. The controls were complaint-free adults (530 females and 2450 males) who volunteered to participate in a stomato-oncological screening in the same period. The age of female patients was especially important in this study. For each interviewed OC woman controls were chosen who matched the patient's age (within 5 months) at the time of cancer diagnosis. The mean age of control male patients was chosen so as to be similar to OC males within 1 year.

Data of the OC patients and their controls were collected through questionnaires and case reports of the inpatients.

Male-female ratio of oral cancer cases. The ratio of male to female OC cases was 3.7:1established on their pooled populations. Male-female ratios were also separately evaluated in different age groups of OC cases; below 30 and above 60 years of age.

The age below 30 means a too short time for exogenous carcinogen exposition to induce clinically diagnosable cancers. The male to female ratio in the small group of patients below 30 years of age showed lower excess of male cases: 1.5:1, with 12 male (0.5%) and 8 female cases (1.5%) in this young age group.

The age above 60 was an appropriate borderline based on the average age of menopause among Hungarian women (or about 50 yrs) to which 10 years were added, as clinical manifestation of tumors requires at least this period from their initiation. Evaluation of the ratio of patients above 60 years of age revealed that 30.2% (643 cases) of male and on the contrary 58.5% (310 cases) of female oral OC cases belonged to this age group. The male to female ratio of this elderly group of patients was 2.1:1, which was significantly lower as compared with that of all patients.

Table 5.1. Mean age of oral cancer (OC) patients and ratio of young and elderly cases

	Males	Females	p
Mean age of all OC cases (yrs)	55.1±10.8 (range:33-85)	63.5±10.9 (range:36-91)	p<0.001
Mean age of gingival cancer cases (yrs)	56.9±11.1	66.9±11.4	p<0.01
Mean age of Sublingual cancer cases (yrs)	54.7±10.9	56.5±10.1	p>0.05
Rate of OC cases <30 yrs	0.5%	1.5%	p<0.05
Rate of OC cases >60 yrs	30.2%	58.5%	p<0.05

Table 5.2. Prevalence of smoking in OC and control cases

	Males			Females		
	Ratio of smokers	p	OR	Ratio of smokers	p	OR
Controls	53.0%			38.3%		
All OC	75.1%	<0.01	3.67	57.2%	<0.01	2.15
Sublingual cancer	84.5%	<0.01	4.80	75.9%	<0.01	5.04
Gingival cancer	68.2%	<0.05	1.89	45.4%	>0.05	1.33

Table 5.3. Correlations between alcohol consumption habits and oral cancer incidence

	All alcohol consumer OC cases		Moderate alcohol consumer OC cases		Excessive alcohol consumer OC cases	
Male OC cases	47.7%		6.6%		41.1%	
Male control cases	21.0%		3.4%		17.6%	
	p<0.01	OR=3.26	p<0.05	OR=2.02	p<0.01	OR=3.44
Female OC cases	12.0%		2.8%		9.2%	
Female control cases	5.5%		2.7%		2.8%	
	p<0.05	OR=2.36	p>0.05 NS	OR=1.00	p<0.01	OR=3.72

Age of patients. (Table 5.1). The mean ages of OC patients were separately evaluated in the male and female groups concerning all patients. The mean age of female OC patients upon admission was significantly higher as compared with the male OC patients. Mean ages of male and female OC cases in the groups of the prevailing tumor locations were also established. The highest mean age was registered among the female gingival cancer cases. In the male gingival cancer group the mean age was moderately elevated as compared with all male OC cases. The lowest mean ages were observed in the sublingual cancer groups both among male and female cases.

Tumor locations. Frequencies of the different tumor locations among the male and female OC cases were compared. Among male OC patients the most common tumor site was the floor of the mouth (41.6%). This was followed in decreasing order by the tongue (24.6%), lower lip (15.3%), gingiva (12.9%), palate (2.5%), bucca (2.1%) and other rare locations (1.0%). In respect to the female patients, the site prevalence was quite different. The most common OC location was the gingiva (28.3%), followed in decreasing order by the floor of the mouth (26.4%), the tongue (18.3%), lower lip (8.4%), bucca (7.1%) palate (6.1%), and other rare locations (0.6%).

Smoking habits. (Table 5.2). Smoking habits and the rate of smokers among the male and female patients with OC and their controls were separately evaluated. In the male OC group the ratio of active smokers and earlier smokers was significantly higher as compared with the male control patients. Among the female oral cancer patients the ratio of smokers was also significantly higher, as compared with the smoking histories of the female control cases.

Mean ages of smokers and non-smokers among the male and female patients at the time of OC diagnosis were evaluated (Table 5.3). Among male OC patients, smokers had a significantly lower mean age as compared with the non-smoker cases. Among female OC cases, smokers exhibited also significantly lower mean age when compared with the female non-smoker OC group.

The rates of smokers were established in the groups with the prevailing OC locations both for the male and female OC cases (Table 5.4). The rate of smokers was the highest in the sublingual cancer subgroups both among the male and female OC cases. Accordingly, tobacco exhibited a high cancer risk to the sublingual mucosa in both genders. The rate of smokers was relatively lower in the gingival cancer groups both among males and females.

Alcohol consumption. (Table 5.5) Regular alcohol consumption among OC and control male patients and among OC and control women was registered within which moderate and excessive drinking was separately evaluated. Regular <25 g/die alcohol intake was regarded as moderate, >25 g/die was regarded as excessive alcohol consumption.

Table 5.4. Prevalence of alcohol consumption in OC and control cases

	Males			Females		
	Ratio of alcohol consumers	p	OR	Ratio of alcohol consumers	p	OR
Controls	21.0%			5.5%		
All OC	47.7%	<0.01	3.26	12.0%	<0.05	2.36
Sublingual cancer	58.1%	<0.01	5.22	20.4%	<0.001	4.46
Gingival cancer	46.7%	<0.01	3.30	11.3%	>0.05	0.93

Table 5.5. Prevalence of elevated fasting glucose (EFG) in oral cancer cases

	Males			Females		
	Ratio of EFG	p	OR	Ratio of EFG	p	OR
Controls	52.5%			43.5%		
All OC	51.9%	>0.05	0.97	55.4%	<0.05	1.61
Sublingual cancer	51.6%	>0.05	0.96	53.7%	<0.05	1.51
Gingival cancer	56.8%	>0.05	19-Jan	56.9%	<0.05	1.69

Table 5.6. History of menopause in the groups of OC and control females

	Sublingua l cancer	Gingival cancer	ALL OC females	Control females	p value
Postmenopausal cases	97.80%	100.00%	98.00%	74.00%	p<0.001
Mean age at menopause	44.50%	47.30%	45,3 yrs	50,9 yrs	p<0.01
Early menopause cases (<45yrs)	29.10%	31.90%	31.40%	16.00%	p<0.05 OR=2.36
Late menopause cases (>45yrs)	13.10%	14.60%	14.30%	23.10%	p<0.05 OR=0.78
Hysterectomy and/or ovarectomy cases	35.20%	33.80%	35.10%	18.40%	p<0.05 OR=1.69

Table 5.7. History of menopause of OC females and controls

	Sublingual cancer	Gingival cancer	ALL OC females	Control females	p value
Postmenopausal cases	97.80%	100.00%	98.00%	74.00%	p<0.001
Mean age at menopause	44.50%	47.30%	45,3 yrs	50,9 yrs	p<0.01
Early menopause cases (<45yrs)	29.10%	31.90%	31.40%	16.00%	p<0.05 OR=2.36
Late menopause cases (>45yrs)	13.10%	14.60%	14.30%	23.10%	p<0.05 OR=0.78
Hysterectomy and/or ovarectomy cases	35.20%	33.80%	35.10%	18.40%	p<0.05 OR=1.69

In the male OC group near half the cases were regular alcohol consumers; with only a small part being moderate drinkers, whereas the majority were excessive drinkers. A significantly lower regular alcohol consumption rate was registered in the male control group with the great majority being excessive drinkers. In men alcohol consumption proved to be a high risk factor for OC, though the risk was lowered among moderate drinkers.

In the female OC group, the rate of regular alcohol consumption was significantly lower as compared with the male OC group. Among the female drinker OC patients the excessive drinkers predominated. Regarding the female control cases, the regular alcohol consumption rate was significantly lower as compared with the female OC cases. Regular excessive alcohol consumption proved also to be a high risk factor for OC among women; however, regular moderate alcohol consumption was not an OC risk for them.

Correlations between drinking and tumor locations were also evaluated in both the male and female OC groups (Table 5.6). Alcohol consumption proved to be a higher risk for sublingual cancer when compared with all OC cases in both genders. Among males with gingival cancer the rate of regular drinkers was similar as compared with all male OC cases. However, among female gingival cancer cases, drinking proved to be a slightly lower risk factor, as compared with all OC women.

Elevated fasting glucose (EFG). (Table 5.7) Ratios of EFG cases among male and female OC and control cases were established. Fasting blood glucose levels were determined repeatedly within 4 days. The level was regarded as elevated only if it was repeatedly >5.5 mmol/l. These EFG groups comprised symptom-free insulin resistant cases, newly diagnosed and known, treated or untreated type-2 diabetes cases.

In the male OC group the EFG rate was quite similar to that of control men. However, among female OC cases EFG proved to be a risk factor as its rate in OC women was significantly higher as compared with that of female controls.

Correlations between EFG rate and tumor location were also studied in the male and female groups. EFG rates of patients in the sublingual and gingival cancer groups were examined separately in both genders because of the primacy of these locations among the male and female OC patients.

The EFG rate in the group of *male sublingual cancer* cases was similar both among the male controls and all male OC cases. EFG proved to be no risk factor for sublingual cancer in men. In contrast, regarding the *female sublingual cancer* cases, the EFG rate was significantly higher as compared with the female controls. EFG was a demonstrable risk factor for sublingual cancer in women.

The EFG rate was found slightly higher in the *male gingival cancer* group as compared with the rate found in controls and with all the male OC patients. EFG proved to be no risk factor for gingival cancer in males. In the *female gingival cancer* group the EFG rate was significantly elevated as compared with the controls and moderately elevated in comparison with all female OC cases. EFG proved to be an even higher risk for gingival cancer in women when compared with all female OC cases.

Menopausal history of the female patients (Table 5.8). The rate of postmenopausal cases and the mean age at menopause in the oral cancer and control groups were established. Female OC patients were near all postmenopausal, whereas a quarter of the control women in the same age group were premenopausal. Mean age at menopause was significantly lower among the female OC patients as compared with the female controls.

Rates of early menopause (<45 yrs) and late menopause (>51 yrs) were also registered both in the oral cancer and control female groups. Rate of early menopause (<45 yrs) due to unidentified ovarian failure or hysterectomy and/or ovarectomy was significantly higher among OC women, as compared with the control patients. Rate of late menopause was significantly lower in the OC group of women as compared with their controls.

Hysterectomy and/or ovarectomy occurred significantly more frequently in the history of female OC cases as compared with the controls.

Mean time-intervals between menopause and oral cancer diagnosis (M-OC) were established for all OC cases and for the early, normal, and late menopausal case groups. The mean M-OC interval among all female OC patients was 16.9 years (range: 3-35 years). The mean M-OC interval in the female OC group with early menopause was significantly lower (13.4 yrs) and in the female OC group with late menopause significantly longer (23.5 yrs) as compared with all OC women ($p<0.05$, and $p<0.05$, respectively).

M-OC intervals of all OC females and separately in the smoker and non-smoker oral cancer patients were established. Mean M-OC intervals related to smoker and non-smoker OC females resulted in significant differences: 11.9 years for smokers and 19.2 years for non-smokers ($p<0.01$).

The rate and length of postmenopausal hormone replacement therapy were also registered. Postmenopausal hormone replacement therapy was relatively rare both in the OC group (8.4 %) and in the control group (10.5%), and showed no significant difference ($p>0.05$). The hormone therapy was relatively short; the mean length was 1.6 yrs in the OC group, and 1.9 yrs in the control group.

Systemic Risk Factors for Oral Cancer

Today the role of insulin resistance in the initiation and progression of cancers is undoubtedly justified (see Chapter 3). However, the role of estrogen deficiency in the development of malignancies is completely obscure. Separated analysis of the well known exogenous and the newly established endogenous OC risk factors in male and female patients yielded striking differences. Apart from the well-known risk of tobacco and alcohol, elevated fasting glucose and postmenopausal sex hormone deficiency in women proved to be strong risk factors affecting OC incidence [62,63].

In our study the male to female ratio of all oral cancer cases was as high as 3.7:1. The male to female ratio of very young cases below 30 years of age and of the elderly patients above 60 years of age exhibited significantly lower values: 1.5 and 2.1, respectively. The latter value revealed an increased accumulation of elderly female cases among oral cancer patients. The highest male to female ratio (4.9:1) was observed among the oral cancer cases between 40 and 60 years of age. Summarizing the gender-related distribution of oral cancer cases, the male to female ratio is low among young cases below 30 years of age, high between 40-60 years of age and exhibits a decline again among elderly cases >60 years of age.

These findings support the assumption that a postmenopausal period longer than 10 years may be associated with an increased risk of clinical manifestation of oral cancer among women. Specific features of the lower male to female ratio among very young and elderly OC cases and the possible explanations will be discussed in Chapter 6.

In the present study, significantly lower incidence of OC among women and higher mean age of female OC patients as compared with males were established. Moreover, the majority of women with OC were older than 60 years, whereas less than one third of OC men belonged to this age group. These results may allow the assumption that women are defended against OC initiation in their reproductive period. The almost exclusively postmenopausal state of the female OC patients and the long mean interval (near 17 yrs) between their menopause and tumor diagnosis also suggested an important role of estrogen deprivation in OC epidemiology. Significantly younger mean age at menopause and considerably higher rate of hysterectomy and/or ovarectomy among the female OC patients in comparison with the control women were also established. These observations suggest that a shorter hormonally active period may be a risk factor for oral cancer among women.

Similarly to our observations, a statistically significant increase of bladder cancer was associated with postmenopausal state and early menopause in female cases [39]. An increased risk for renal cell carcinoma was also reported among women who were subjected to hysterectomy with or without oophorectomy [8]. These observations also support the correlations between estrogen deficiency and cancer risk.

Elevated fasting glucose is an easily accessible mirror to reflect the different stages of the glucose metabolism disorder with the exception of the early hyperinsulinemic phases. The results of the present study underline that EFG is a strong risk factor for OC in estrogen deficient postmenopausal women, especially in cases with gingival cancer. In contrast, among male OC patients EFG is not a marked risk factor.

This gender related difference was also observed in a prospective study, which resulted in a close association between hyperglycemia and increased total cancer risk in women, but not in men [60]. Unfortunately the menopausal history of these women was not available.

Oral mucosa and especially the gingiva are thoroughly affected by hormonal influences [40]. Type-2 diabetes is associated with increased prevalence of gingivitis and periodontitis in both genders. Moreover, in postmenopausal women reduced estrogen level results in atrophic, desquamative gingivitis.

In the present study the conspicuous difference of the prevailing OC locations between male and female patients supplied a further key to reveal the gender specific risks.

Among the female OC patients the gingiva was the most prominent tumor location (28.3%), however in the male OC group gingival cancer incidence was significantly lower (13.0%). In the female gingival cancer group, EFG proved to be a stronger risk factor as compared with all OC women. Exogenous carcinogenic noxae (alcohol and tobacco) could not be demonstrated in near one third of the male and in more than half of the female gingival cancer group! These results suggest that a combined estrogen deficiency and insulin resistance may play etiologic role in gingival cancer development among postmenopausal women, even in the absence of traditional exogenous cancer risk factors.

Primacy of sublingual cancers among male OC patients may be explained by the higher rate of smoking and alcohol consumption as compared with the OC women. These well-known carcinogenic noxae are dissolved and concentrated in the saliva of the floor of the mouth resulting in strong, local carcinogenic effect. However, smoking and excessive alcohol consumption means double cancer risks for the oral mucosa by means of their local toxic derivatives and systemic metabolic effects.

Alcohol consumption is a well-known, strong risk factor for OC. However, mild to moderate alcohol consumption is associated with improved insulin sensitivity and advantageous metabolic impact, while the two extremes: complete abstinence and excessive drinking are risks for insulin resistance in both genders. In postmenopausal women, regular moderate alcohol consumption mediates the increase of insulin sensitivity and estrogen synthesis in the peripheral adipose tissue (see Chapter 2).

In our study, excessive alcohol consumption proved to be a high risk for OC both in the male and female cases. Among male patients moderate alcohol intake was a lower OC risk as compared with heavy drinkers. Presumably, the local effects of toxic metabolites on the oral mucosa may be antagonized by the advantageous systemic, metabolic impact. However, in postmenopausal women moderate drinking was not an OC risk factor at all, which may be attributed to both increased insulin sensitivity and elevated estrogen level.

In this study smoking was a high risk for oral cancer both among men and women in concordance with the results of earlier studies (see Chapter 1). On the other hand, smoking seemed to be an anticipating factor for OC initiation in the groups of both male and female OC patients as the mean age of smokers was significantly lower as compared with the non-smoker cases.

The highest rates of non-smoker cases were found in the gingival cancer groups both among male and female OC patients. Near one third (29.4%) of the male group and more than half (54.5%) of the female group with gingival cancers were registered as non-smoker cases. These findings suggest that strongly gender-related factors may have a role in gingival cancer risk among non-smoker OC patients. Correlations among smoking, insulin resistance and changes in the sexual hormone levels are discussed in Chapter 2 and 8.

Summarizing the presented results, early menopause, postmenopausal state and fairly long interval between menopause and tumor onset proved to be significantly high cancer risk factors among female oral cancer cases. These results strongly suggest a role of estrogen deficiency in oral cancer incidence [62,63].

Estrogen Deficiency as Cancer Risk

The new theory of estrogen deficiency as cancer risk factor is not a simple negation of the traditional concept concerning the carcinogenic capacity of estrogen, but means a complete conversion. It is a fairly heretical idea that no estrogen but its deficiency may provoke cancer initiation.

This new hypothesis may explain the conspicuously lower oral cancer incidence among middle aged female cases as they have a hormonal defense during their reproductive period. The significantly older age of women with oral cancer as compared with men may be attributed to the postmenopausal estrogen deficiency, which may initiate mutations in the perimenopausal years or later. Development of clinically observable tumors requires many years after menopause resulting in an accumulation of cancers among elderly women.

This new theory supplies some explanation to the mystery of oral cancer incidence among non-smoker, non-drinker elderly women and the unique characteristics of oral cancer epidemiology among young cases (see Chapter 8). The decreasing trend of the earlier very high male to female ratio of oral cancer may be at least partially attributed to the globally increased prevalence of type-2 diabetes (see Chapter 2) and its greater impact on oral cancer risk among women as compared with men. The causal correlation between estrogen deficiency and cancer initiation may also clarify many controversial associations of female sexual steroids and malignancies and justifies the role of estrogen in female longevity.

This novel hypothesis of estrogen deficiency and elevated fasting glucose as systemic risk factors for OC may provide new insights into the etiology of oral malignancies. Moreover, it may reveal new possibilities in prevention and treatment of oral cancer and open a pathway to new strategies for cancer research.

Molecular Mechanisms of Estrogen Action

The most potent and dominant estrogen hormone in humans is estradiol, but other hormones with estrogen effect are estrone and estriol exhibited in lower concentrations. Both theories on cancer provoking effect and anticancer capacity of estrogen require justifications at cellular level.

The roles of estrogen and its receptors in gene regulation are thoroughly studied [2,3,6,54]. However, many of the researches reflect bias to estrogen carcinogenicity in spite of their valuable results. A review of unbiased literary data on molecular mechanism of estrogen action suggests that estrogen orchestrates the gene regulation of cell proliferation with high safety. Cross talk of estrogen receptors with other hormonal and growth factor signals, their agonistic and antagonistic interplay with other gene regulators suggest an indispensable role of estrogen in cell biology. However, estrogen deficiency may elicit a breakdown of the exquisite surveillance of gene regulation and results in cancer initiation beyond retrieval.

Gene regulation mechanisms affected by estrogen have a fairly wide range during embryonic growth, development and differentiation, and have a crucial role in the hormonal and metabolic processes both in males and females throughout life. Estrogen, based on its pivotal role in gene regulation, has been accused of its carcinogenicity. However, as estrogen is a proven commander in chief in the regulation of the endocrine system, metabolism, and cell proliferation an extreme safeguarding is necessary to have domination over these highly responsible mechanisms.

Estrogen Receptors and Their Actions

In 1962 an estrogen binding receptor protein had been identified from rat uterus, which was supposed to mediate all actions of estrogen [16]. More than three decades later, in 1996 another isoform of estrogen receptor (ER) was discovered and named as ER-β [26], whereas the former ER was renamed as ER-α. These ER isoforms are the products of two distinct genes located on distinct chromosomes [7].

ERs belong to the steroid-thyroid hormone nuclear receptor superfamily [43]. The classic, genomic mechanism of ER action is that estrogen binding activates ERs in the nucleus and they act as transcriptional modulators by binding to specific sequences in the promoter region of target genes [3,10]. However, other signaling pathways that deviate from the classical model have been discovered, and recently it has been accepted that ERs regulate gene expression by a number of distinct mechanisms [3] (Figure 5.1).

ERs can also regulate gene expression without direct binding to DNA, which occurs through interactions between receptor protein and other DNA-binding transcription factor proteins in the nucleus [3]. This interaction between ERs and transcription factors may result in either stimulation or inhibition in gene transcription processes [43]. Moreover, by means of some not clearly identified mechanisms, ERs may regulate the expression of genes that do not contain estrogen responsive elements (EREs).

Evidences are accumulating that estrogen action have also non-genomic, membrane associated signaling cascades [54]. Non-genomic actions may influence both protein functions as cytoplasmic network of coordination and regulation of gene expression in the nucleus. Non-genomic actions are exerted by membrane associated ERs. Controversial concepts have been published concerning the nature of ERs located at the plasma membrane. Some authors have suggested that the non-genomic estrogen effects are mediated through a subpopulation of the classical two ER isoforms [49].

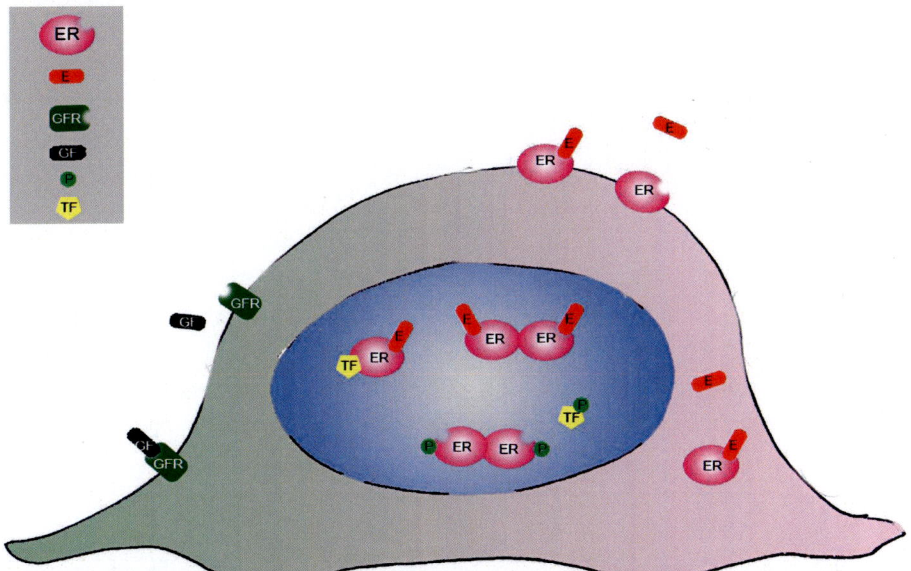

Schematic picture of Estrogen Receptor and Growth Factor Receptor actions
ER - Estrogen Receptor; E - Estrogen; GFR - Growth Factor Receptor; - GF - Growth Factor
P - Phosphate; TF - Transforming Factor

Source: Björnström L and Sjöberg M, Molecular Endocrinology 19:833-842, 2005

Figure 5.1 Schematic Illustration of ER Signaling Mechanisms 1. Classical mechanism of ER action. Nuclear E2-ERs bind directly to EREs in target gene promoters. 2. ERE-independent genomic actions. Nuclear E2-ER complexes are tethered through protein-protein interactions to a transcription factor complex (TF) that contacts the target gene promoter. 3. Ligand-independent genomic actions. Growth factors (GF) activate protein-kinase cascades, leading to phosphorylation (P) and activation of nuclear ERs at EREs. 4. Nongenomic actions. Membrane E2-ER complexes activate protein-kinase cascades, leading to altered functions of proteins in the cytoplasm, *e.g.* activation of eNOS, or to regulation of gene expression through phosphorylation (P) and activation of a TF.

Finally, genomic and non-genomic pathways of estrogen receptor signaling converge on the target genes [3]. Several signal transduction pathways may connect the non-genomic estrogen actions to genomic responses. Many nuclear transcription factors are regulated through non-genomic protein kinase mediated phosphorylation, and these transcription factors may thus become targets for non-genomic estrogen actions. This complex signaling system provides exquisitely safety control and plasticity of tissue responses to estrogen and also contributes to the divergence of tissue-specific actions [54].

ER-α is widely expressed throughout the female genital organs, such uterus, vagina, ovaries and mammary glands, whereas it is also highly exhibited in the brain, bone, liver and cardiovascular system [20].

ER-β is also widely distributed throughout the body. It has been shown to be the dominant isoform in the prostate, testis, salivary glands, ovary, vascular endothelium, smooth muscle, certain neurons and cells of the immune system [23]. Estrogen receptors in the immune competent cells enable estrogen to regulate defense mechanisms against inflammatory processes, infections, shock and even malignant transformation.

Some tissues, such as mammary glands, uterus, brain, bone and cardiovascular system express both ER isoforms, with the predominance of one or the other [23,43]. Surprisingly, all these sites are especially endangered in estrogen deficient, postmenopausal women. Incidence of ischemic attacks in the central nervous system, osteoporosis and dyslipidemic cardiovascular diseases is conspicuously increased in estrogen deficient female cases after menopause. In these diseases estrogen therapy has more or less beneficial effects, especially in the initial phases. Dangers of estrogen loss related to the breast and endometrium are discussed in Chapters 6 and 7.

The presence of both alpha and beta ER isoforms was confirmed in adipocytes deriving from the subcutaneous and intra-abdominal fat with evident predominance of ER-α [5]. Fatty tissue accumulation is fairly dependent on the balance of sexual steroid levels. Estrogen tends to promote the gluteofemoral fat deposition [25], whereas loss of estrogen and androgen excess is associated with abdominal obesity and strongly increases the risk of insulin resistance [48].

Postmenopausal aromatase activity and estrogen production in the adipose tissue have important role in many biological processes [17]. Recently, adipocytes have been regarded as endocrine cells. Fatty tissue is hormone dependent and in animal models hormones and cytokines produced by adipocytes have actions in remote organs, such as liver, muscle, bone, central nervous system and others [38]. Human adipose tissue and its secreted products have important role in the hormonal and metabolic processes. Hormonal regulation of human adipocytes may serve as a cross road among obesity, hypertension and insulin resistance [64].

Different actions of ER-α and ER-β were observed on neuroblastoma cells transfected with either ER-α or ER-β. Activation of ER-α caused an increase in length and number of neurites, whereas ER-β activation resulted only in neurite elongation [44].

Discovery of selective agonists for ER-α and ER-β brought new possibilities to research the specificity of estrogen receptors. In an epithelial cell line obtained from pregnant mouse mammary glands both ER-α and ER-β were expressed. It was observed that selective agonists for ER-α provoke cell proliferation and agonists for ER-β inhibit cell growth on this in vitro model [12]. These findings suggest that functional equilibrium of the two receptor isoforms may supply excellent surveillance for cell growth and differentiation.

Development of the three knockout mouse lines: estrogen receptor-α and β knockout (ER-αKO, ER-βKO) [24] and aromatase enzyme knockout (ARKO) mice provided new opportunities for understanding the individual actions of the two estrogen receptors and of estrogen itself. In vivo studies on these knockout mice have demonstrated that ER-α and ER-β may have distinct, even opposite effects. Development of distinct autoimmune diseases in different knockout mice revealed that ER-α and ER-β have specific functions in the maintenance of the normal immune system [2,55,56].

In addition to the specific function of each receptor, interplay between these two receptor isoforms has been reported when they are coexpressed. ER-β may oppose ER-α-mediated activity in many systems, moreover, ER-α and ER-β together may elicit completely opposite responses in the presence of estradiol [10,35]. In ER-βKO mice, ER-α-mediated gene expression was increased by 85% as compared with animals expressing both receptors. This observation suggested that ER-β in normal mice reduces ER-α-regulated gene transcription, supporting the idea of a "ying yang" relationship between the two receptors [29].

However, considering the magnitude, complexity and safety of estrogen receptor signals, actions of ER-α and ER-β can be hardly imagined as a mechanical equilibrium of a seesaw. Though there are multiple cross talks and interplays between the two ER isoforms, they don't keep each other on leash rather, both of them may have their autoregulation with simultaneous feed back control of the actions of each other. ER knockout mice are artificially disabled animals and similar disorders may occur extremely rarely as spontaneous mutations. Unexpected, increased gene expression elicited by the singly remaining ER-α may probably be attributed to an emergency substitution of the action of the missing ER-β isoform.

ERs display similar DNA- and ligand binding properties in vitro, however, ER-β shows lower transcriptional activity than ER-α. Experimental results revealed that in the absence of estradiol both type of ERs interacted with estrogen responsive elements (EREs) of the nucleus similarly. However, estradiol application enhanced the ERE binding of ER-α but not that of ER-β. Thus, the interaction between ER-β and ERE seemed to be independent of estradiol and could be impaired by its amino terminus [15]. These findings provided additional explanation for differences between ER-α and ER-β actions. Moreover, these data also reveal that estrogen loss may yield thorough changes in gene expression mechanisms.

Summarizing the literary data, estradiol action depends on the ratio of receptor isoforms expressed in the given tissue. Moreover, in case of coexpression of the two receptors interactions of their signaling pathways will variably modulate the transcription of target genes [2]. The great variations in tissular distribution and isoform predominance of ERs have been a source of intense debate among researchers. However, a widely accepted concept is that though ER-α and ER-β have distinct biological functions supposedly they act in a close interplay.

These overwhelming routes of estrogen effects and ER actions support that estrogen may use many different signaling pathways and will evoke distinct gene responses depending on the types of target cells and on the nature of temporary intra- and extracellular stimuli [3].

Actions of Estrogen and ERs on Nonclassical Target Tissues

Hormonal effects on the classical endocrine target organs of the female reproductive system have been thoroughly studied both on cell cultures and experimental animal models. However, estrogens have widespread, beneficial actions in nonclassical target tissues as well.

Results of clinical and epidemiological findings suggest that estrogens and their receptors have pivotal role in health maintenance of the cardiovascular, immune competent and neuroendocrine system, as well as in the gastrointestinal tract and liver [41]. Estrogen signal maintains the equilibrium of glucose and lipid metabolism by several pathways [2,67], reduces the oxidative stress [66] and regulates the maintenance of fluid and electrolyte homeostasis [59]. In aged male rats estrogen exhibited an anti-aging effect by means of a decreased lipid peroxidation and improvement of the parameters of liver dysfunction [11].

Estrogen has not only preventive but also curing effects on diseases of the vasculature. Estradiol may contribute to the vascular healing process and prevention of restenosis by interplay of both ERs. Through ERα activation estradiol may induce reendothelization and through ERβ stimulation inhibits migration and proliferation of smooth muscle cells in the vessel wall [9].

Cross Talk between Receptor Signals of Estrogen and Growth Factors

Non-genomic actions of estrogen are too rapid to be attributed to activation of RNA and protein synthesis. These actions are common properties of steroid hormones and are frequently associated with activation of various protein-kinase cascades [30]. By these ways ERs have thorough surveillance on cell proliferation, which is their basic function during growth, differentiation and whole cell life.

Membrane associated ERs may activate membrane tyrosine kinase receptors in various cell types. ER-α activated by estradiol interacts directly with the IGF-I receptor, leading to its activation [65], and hence activation of the mitogen associated protein kinase (MAPK) signaling pathway [18]. These data demonstrate that estradiol activated ER-α is required for rapid activation of the IGF-IR signaling cascade.

Estradiol liganded ERs in the plasma membrane can rapidly stimulate signal transductions that are G-protein coupled. This was reported to occur through the transactivation of the epidermal growth factor receptor (EGFR) or insulin-like growth factor-I receptor (IGF-IR) [50]. Estrogen can over regulate the IGF-I gene transcription by involving an AP-I enhancer [65].

Estrogen signaling is coupled to growth factor signaling with a feedback mechanism directly impacting function of growth factor receptors [6]. ER signaling pathways involving specific complexes of cytoplasmic proteins might quench or augment the growth factor activities! On the other hand, the mitogen activated protein kinase system (MAPK) is capable of phosphorylation of human estrogen receptor in vitro, and in cells treated with epidermal growth factor (EGF) and insulin like growth factor (IGF) in vivo. Thus activity of the amino-terminal AF-l of ER may be modulated by the phosphorylation of Ser118 via the Ras-MAPK cascade of the growth factor signaling pathways [19].

Studies in rodents have shown that EGF is able to mimic the uterotropic effects of estrogen suggesting a physiological coupling of growth factor and steroid receptor signaling pathways. These results supplied a "cross-talk" model in which EGF receptor signaling resulted in activation of nuclear ERs [42]. However, in ER knockout mice epidermal growth factor could not elicit an estrogen-like response, which revealed that intact ERs are necessary for the activation of ER target genes by growth factors [4].

Estrogen has a crucial role in regulation of growth hormone receptor (GHR) activities as well [28]. Estrogen attenuates growth hormone (GH) action by means of inhibition of its secretion and suppression of cellular GHR functions. Estrogen and GH concentrations are strongly correlated during puberty and later, in adult life GH levels are regularly higher in women than in men. In man the stimulatory effect of androgens on GH secretion depends on the ratio of their prior aromatisation to estrogens. All these observations suggest that estrogens play a major and positive role in the regulation of GH-IGF-I axis in both genders [28], which may be in close correlation with their antidiabetogenic and anticancer capacities.

Estrogen Receptors and Human Cancers

There are literary data on the supposed roles of estrogen and membrane-associated ER signaling pathways in human cancer induction [13,47], particularly in breast cancer cases [22,33,45].

Interactions of estrogen and growth factor receptors have been recently revealed in breast, lung and cholangial cancers [1,46]. In the majority of in vitro experiments on different tumor cell lines a close synergism of expressed estrogen and growth factor receptors was supposed in the modulation of cell growth and proliferation.

Estrogen treatment could inhibit lung carcinogenesis by reducing levels of IGF-I [34], which is a potent mitogenic agent for several malignancies, including lung cancer. These results suggest an alternative role of estrogen and growth factor actions on tumor cell proliferation.

A role of estrogens in the development of lung cancer has been suggested as ERs were demonstrated in non-small cell lung cancers. In recent studies a favorable prognosis for patients with non-small cell lung cancer was established, when tumor cells exhibited increased expression of Erβ [58,68]. Similarly, the absence of Erβ nuclear staining correlated with poor survival in both men and women with lung cancer [21]. Associations of increased ERβ expression with better prognosis of non-small cell lung cancer suggest an anticancer capacity of estrogen signal and raise the idea of beneficial effect of estrogen administration. This assumption seems to be justified by a recent study, which established a significant correlation between hormone replacement therapy and reduced lung cancer risk in postmenopausal women [51].

Highly expressed epidermal growth factor receptors were demonstrated in a variety of solid tumors, including oral cancer, and their activity enhanced the tumor growth and invasive capacity [14]. However, estrogen receptor expression in oral cancers showed no correlation either with tumor progression or with mortality of patients [31]. These results suggest an alternative role of estrogen and growth factor activities in oral cancers.

Inhibition of vascular endothelial growth factor expression by ER-α was exhibited in HEClA endometrial cancer cell line [61]. This finding suggests that inhibition of capillary proliferation in tumors may also be an important part of the anticancer capacity of ERs.

Aromatase inhibitors, which lower the estrogen ligand for ER and pure ER antagonists, which destroy the receptor, are used to cure breast cancer. Recently, recognition of a dynamic, inverse relationship between the expression of ERs and growth factor receptors has brought more excitement. Potential restoring of ER expression in apparently ER-negative breast cancer cells emerged by inhibition of growth factor signaling to overcome resistance to endocrine therapy [36,37]. Abandonment of estrogen deprivation and antiestrogen therapy in breast cancer cases should be more advantageous instead of the idea of combined antiestrogen and anti-growth factor therapy.

The estrogen receptor signal is thoroughly defended from changes of serum estrogen levels by compensatory feedback mechanisms even in tumors. This suggests that elevated estrogen level may hardly produce gene alterations. Excessive estradiol treatment decreased the ER protein quantity in MCF-7 human breast cancer cell line within a few hours [52]. Similarly, estrogen administration evoked a decrease in ER-α protein and estrogen responsiveness in rat pituitaries [53]. However, in experimental animals the low serum estrogen levels increased the mRNA level of ERs [57].

This strict feedback regulation suggests that overexpression of ERs in highly differentiated tumor cells means an increased estrogen demand induced by estrogen deficiency rather than defense against excessive hormone supply. Considering that actions of the ER signal are not dangerous but represent the highest control on gene regulation, estrogen administration may improve the disturbances of cell growth and proliferation in receptor-positive tumor cells.

Estrogen and growth factors are potent mitogenic stimuli that share important, competitive capacities in the control of cell proliferation. Cross talk between ER and growth factor signals assures a finical equilibrium and may result in either synergistic or antagonistic effects on gene regulation. Exquisitely organized genomic and non-genomic actions of ERs and their convergence on the target genes rather serve as defense of gene regulation with safety surveillance of multitude players of cell biology than as risk for malignancy.

In the absence of estrogens, the biological equilibrium of gene regulation is endangered. There is no estrogen to exert its indispensable, beneficial cellular actions and to oppose overwhelming growth factor activities. Accumulation of non-liganded ERs in an estrogen deficient milieu may also result in accidental coupling of ER and GF signals. Moreover, IGF-I and EGF signaling pathways can modulate the functions of exposed, non-liganded ERs through phosphorylation of the receptors on certain residues [6]. These might be dangerous processes as unopposed growth factor activities and altered phosphorylation of non-liganded ERs may provoke a blunder in gene regulation of cell proliferation. Breakdown in the main regulatory signals may result in cancer initiation. Discovery of estrogen deficiency as a tumor-inducing factor is knocking at the door.

References

[1] Alvaro D, Barbaro B, Franchitto A, Onori P, Glaser SS, Alpini G, Francis H, Marucci L, Sterpetti P, Ginanni-Corradini S, Onetti MA, Dostal DE, De Santis A, Attili AF, Benedetti A, Gaudio E: Estrogens and insulin-like growth factor I modulate neoplastic cell growth in human cholangiocarcinoma. *Am. J. Path* 169:877-888, 2006

[2] Barros RPA, Machado UF, Gustafsson JA: Estrogen receptors: new players in diabetes mellitus. *Trends in Molecular Medicine* 9: 425-431, 2006

[3] Björnström L, Sjöberg M: Mechanisms of estrogen receptor signaling: Convergence of genomic and nongenomic actions on target genes. *Molecular Endocrinology* 19:833-842, 2005

[4] Curtis SW, Washburn T, Sewall C, DiAugustine R, Lindzey J, Couse JF et al: Physiological coupling of growth factor and steroid receptor signaling pathway: estrogen receptor knockout mice lack estrogen-like response to epidermal growth factor. *Proceed Natl. Acad. Sci. USA* 93: 12626-12630, 1996

[5] Dieudonne MN, et al: Evidence for functional estrogen receptors α and β in human adipose cells: regional specipities and regulation by estrogens. *Am. J. Physiol. Cell Physiol.* 286:C655-C661, 2004

[6] Driggers PH, Segars JH: Estrogen action and cytoplasmic signaling pathways. Part II: The role of growth factors and phosphorylation in estrogen signaling. *Trends Endocrin. Metab.* 13:422-427, 2002

[7] Enmark E, Pelto-Huikko M, Grandien K, Lagercrantz S, Lagercrantz J, Fried G, Nordenskjold M, Gustafsson JA: Human estrogen receptor beta-gene structure, chromosomal localization and expression pattern. *J. Clin. Endocrinol. Metab.* 82:4258-4265, 1997

[8] Gago-Domingez M, Castelao JE, Yuan JM, Ross RK, Yu MC: Increased Risk of Renal Cell Carcinoma Subsequent to Hysterectomy. *Cancer Epidemiology, Biomarkers and Prevencion* 8: 999-1003, 1999

[9] Geraldes P, Sirois MG, Tanguay JF: Specific contribution of estrogen receptors on mitogen-activated protein kinase pathways and vascular cell activation. *Circ. Res.* 93: 399-405, 2003

[10] Hall JM, and McDonnell DP: The estrogen receptor β-isoform (ERβ) of the human estrogen receptor modulates ERα transcriptional activity and is a key regulator of the cellular response to estrogens and antiestrogens. *Endocrinology* 140:5566-5578, 1999

[11] Hamden K, Carreau S, Ellouz F, Masmoudi H, El FA: Protective effect of 17beta-estradiol on oxidative stress and liver dysfunction in aged male rats. *J. Physiol. Biochem.* 63:195-201, 2007

[12] Helguero LA et al: Estrogen receptors α (ERα) and β (ERβ) differentially regulate proliferation and apoptosis of the normal murine mammary epithelial cell line HC11. *Oncogene* 24:6605-6616, 2005

[13] Henderson BE, Ross R, Bernstein L: Estrogens as a cause of human cancer. *Cancer Res.* 48:246-253, 1988

[14] Hirashi Y, Wada T, Nakatani K, Negoro K, Fujita Sh: Immunohistochemical expression of EGFR and p-EGFR in oral squamous cell carcinomas. *Pathol. Oncol. Res*. 12: 87-91, 2006

[15] Huang J, Li X, Maguire CA, Hilf R, Bambara RA, Muyan M: Binding of estrogen receptor beta to estrogen response element in situ is independent of estradiol and impaired by its amino terminus. *Mol. Endocrinol*. 19:2696-2712, 2005

[16] Jensen EV, Jacobson HI: Basic guides to the mechanism of estrogen action. *Recent Prog. Horm. Res*. 18:387-414, 1962

[17] Judd HI, Shamonki IM, Frumar AM, Lagasse LD: Origin of serum estradiol in postmenopausal women. *Obstet Gynecol*. 59:680-686, 1982

[18] Kahlert S, Neudling S, van Eickels M, Vetter H, Meyer R, Groche C: Estrogen receptor α rapidly activates the IGF-1 receptor pathway. *J. Biol. Chem*. 275:18447-18453, 2000

[19] Kato S, Endoh H, Masuhiro Y, Kitamoto T, Uchiyama S, Sasaki H, Masushige S, Gotoh Y, Nishida E, Kawashima H, Metzger D, Chambon P: Activation of the estrogen receptor though phosphorylation by mitogen-activated protein kinase. *Science* 270: 1491-1494, 1995

[20] Katzenellenbogen BS: Estrogen receptors: bioactivities and interactions with cell signaling pathways. *Biol. Reprod*. 54:287-293, 1996

[21] Kaway H, Ishii A, Washiya K, Konno T, Kon H, Yamaya C, Ono I, Minamiya Y, Ogawa J: Estrogen receptor alpha and beta are prognostic factors in non-small cell lung cancer. *Clin. Cancer Res*. 11:5084-5089, 2005

[22] Key TJ, Applyby PN, Reeves GK et al: Body mass index, serum sex hormones and breast cancer risk in postmenopausal *women. J. Natl. Cancer Inst*. 95:1218-1226, 2003

[23] Koehler KF, et al: Reflections on the discovery and significance of estrogen receptor β. *Endocr. Rev*. 26:465-478, 2005

[24] Krege JK, et al: Generation and reproductive phenotypes of mice lacking estrogen receptor β. *Proc. Natl. Acad.Sci. U.S.A* 95:15677-15682, 1998

[25] Krotkiewski M, Bjorntorp P, Sjostrom et al: Impact of obesity on metabolism in men and women, importance of regional adipose tissue distribution. *J. Clin. Invest* 72:1150-1162, 1983

[26] Kuiper GG et al: Cloning of a novel receptor expressed in rat prostate and ovary. *Proc. Natl. Acad. Sci. USA* 93:5925-5930, 1996

[27] Kumar V, Abbas AK, Fausto N, Mitchell RN: Robbins Basic Pathology. 8th Edition Saunders Elsevier 2007

[28] Leung KC, Johannson G, Leong GM, Ho KKY: Estrogen regulation of growth hormone action. *Endocrine Rev*. 25:693-721, 2004

[29] Lindberg MK.et al: Estrogen receptor (ER)-β reduces ERα-regulated gene transcription, supporting a 'ying yang' relationship between ERα and ERβ in mice. *Mol. Endocrinol*.17:203-208, 2003

[30] Losel R, Wehling M: Nongenomic actions of steroid hormones. *Nat. Rev. Mol. Cell. Biol*. 4:46-56, 2003

[31] Lukits J, Remenar E, Raso E, Ladányi A, Kasler M, Timar J: Molecular identification, expression and prognostic role of estrogen- and progesterone receptors in head and neck cancer. *Int. J. Oncol*. 30:155-160, 2007

[32] Marquez DC, Lee J, Lin T, Pietras RJ: Epidermal growth factor receptor and tyrosine phosphorylation of estrogen receptor. *Endocrine* 16:73-81, 2001a

[33] Marquez DC, Pietras RJ: Membrane-associated binding sites for estrogen contribute to growth regulation in human breast cancer cells. *Oncogene* 20:5420-5430, 2001b

[34] Marquez-Garban DC, Chen HW, Fishbein MC, Goodglick L, Pietras RJ: Estrogen receptor signaling pathways in human non-small cell lung cancer. *Steroids* 72:135-143, 2007

[35] Maruyama S. et al: Suppression by estrogen receptor β of AP-1 mediated transactivation through estrogen receptor α. *J. Steroid Biochem. Mol. Biol.* 78:177-184, 2001

[36] Massarweh S, Schiff R: Resistance to endocrine therapy in breast cancer: exploiting estrogen receptor/growth factor crosstalk. *Endocrin.-Related Cancer Suppl.* 13, 1:S15-24, 2006

[37] Massarweh S, Osborne CK, Creighton CJ, Qin L, Tsimelson A, Huang S, Weiss H, Rimawi M, Schiff R: Tamoxifen resistance in breast tumors is driven by growth factor receptor signaling with repression of classic estrogen receptor genomic function. *Cancer Res.* 68:826-833, 2008

[38] Mattison R, Jensen M: The adipocyte as an endocrine cell. *Curr. Opin. Endocrinol. Diabetes* 10:317-321, 2003

[39] McGrath M, Michaud DS, De Vivo I: Hormonal and reproductive factors and the risk of bladder cancer in women. *Am. J. Epidemiol.* 163: 236-244, 2006

[40] Mealey BL, Moritz AJ: Hormonal influences: effects of diabetes mellitus and endogenous female sex steroid hormones on the periodontium. *Periodontology* 2000. 32:59-81, 2003

[41] Murphy E, Korach KS: Action of estrogen and estrogen receptors on nonclassical target tissues. Ernst Schering Foundation Symposium Proceedings 1:13-24, 2006

[42] Nelson KG, Takahashi T, Bossert NL, Walmer DK, McLachlan JA. CIM. *Proc. Natl. Acad. Sci. USA* 88:21-25, 1991

[43] Nilsson S, Makela S, Treuter E, Tujague J, Thomsen J, Andersson G, Enmark E, Pettersson K, Warner M, Gustafsson JA: Mechanisms of estrogen action. *Physiol. Rev.* 81:1535-1565, 2001

[44] Patrone C. et al: Estradiol induces differential neuronal phenotypes by activating estrogen receptor α or β. *Endocrinology* 141:1839-1845, 2000

[45] Pietras RJ, Arboleda J, Wongvipat N, Ramos L, Parker MG, Sliwkowski MX et al: HER-2 tyrosine kinase pathway targets estrogen receptor and promotes hormone independent growths in human breast cancer cells. *Oncogene* 10:2435-2446, 1995

[46] Pietras RJ, Marquez D, Chen HW, Tsai E, Weinberg O, Fishbein M: Estrogen and growth factor receptor interactions in human breast and non-small cell lung cancer cells. *Steroids* 70:372-381, 2005

[47] Pietras RJ, Marquez-Garban DC: Membrane-associated estrogen receptor signaling pathways in human cancers. *Clin. Cancer Res.* 13:4672-4676, 2007

[48] Poehiman ET, Toth MJ, Gardner AW: Changes in energy balance and body composition at menopause: a controlled longitudinal study. *Ann. Intern. Med.* 123:673-675, 1995 ?

[49] Razandi M, Pedram A, Greene GL, Levin ER: Cell membrane and nuclear estrogen receptors (ERs) originate from a single transcript: studies of ERα and ERβ expressed in Chinese hamster ovary cells. *Mol. Endocrinol.* 13:307-319, 1999

[50] Razandi M, Pedram A, Park ST, Levin ER, Oh P, Schnitzer J: Proximal events in signaling by plasma membrane estrogen receptors ERs associate with and regulate the production of caveolin: implications for signaling and cellular actions. *J. Biol. Chem.* 278:2701-2712, 2003

[51] Rodriguez C, Feigelson HS, Deka A, Patel AV, Jacobs EJ, Thun MJ, Calle EE: Postmenopausal hormone therapy and lung cancer risk in the Cancer Prevention Study II Nutrition Cohort. *Cancer Epidemiol. Biomark and Prev.* 17:655-660, 2008

[52] Saceda M, Lippman ME, Chambon P, Lindsey RL, Ponglikitmongkol M, Puente M, Martin MB: Regulation of the estrogen receptor in MCF-7 cells by estradiol. *Molecular Endocrinology* 2:1157-1162, 1988

[53] Schreihofer DA, Stoler MH, Shupnik MA: Differential expression and regulation of estrogen receptors (ERs) in rat pituitary and cell lines: estrogen decreases ER-(alpha)-protein and estrogen responsiveness. *Endocrinology* 141:2174-2184, 2000

[54] Segars J, Driggers P: Estrogen action and cytoplasmic signaling cascades. Part I: Membrane-associated signaling complexes. *Trends Endocrin. Metab.* 13:349-354, 2002

[55] Shim GJ, et al: Autoimmune glomerulonephritis with spontaneous formation of splenic germinal centers in mice lacking the estrogen receptor α gene. *Proc. Natl. Acad. Sci. USA* 101:1720-1724, 2004a

[56] Shim GJ, et al: Aromatase-deficient mice spontaneously develop a lymphoproliferative autoimmune disease resembling Sjogren's syndrome. *Proc. Natl. Acad. Sci. USA* 101:12628-12633, 2004b

[57] Shupnik MA, Gordon MS, Chin WW: Tissue-specific regulation of rat estrogen receptor mRNAs. *Molecular Endocrinology* 3:660-665, 1989

[58] Skov BG, Fischer BM, Pappot H: Oestrogen receptor beta over expression in males with non-small cell lung cancer is associated with better survival. *Lung Cancer* 59:88-94, 2008

[59] Sladek C, Somponpun SJ: Estrogen receptors: their roles in regulation of vasopressin release for maintenance of fluid and electrolite homeostasis. *Front Neuroendocrin.* 29:114-127, 2008

[60] Stattin P, Bjor O, Ferrari P, Lukanova A, Lenner P, Lindahl B, Hallmans G, Kaaks R: Prospective study of hyperglycemia and cancer risk. *Diabetes Care* 30:561-567, 2007

[61] Stoner M, Wang F, Wormke M, Nguyen T, Samudio I, Vyhlidal C, Marme D, Finkenzeller G, Safe S: Inhibition of vascular endothelial growth factor expression in HEC1A endometrial cancer cells through interactions of estrogen receptor alpha and Sp3 proteins. *J. Biol. Chem.* 275:22769-22779, 2000

[62] Suba Zs: Gender-related hormonal risk factors for oral cancer. *Pathol. Oncol. Res.* 13:195-202, 2007

[63] Suba Zs: Systemic risk factors for oral cancer: Estrogen deficiency and insulin resistance. Chapter 8. pp. 157-172 In: Progress in Oral Cancer Research. Eds: Frederik L. Nielsen. Nova Science Publishers. 2008

[64] Tikhonoff V, Staessen JA: Hormonal regulation of human adipocytes at the cross roads between obesity and hypertension. *J. Hypertens.* 20:839-841, 2002

[65] Umayahara Y, Kawamori R, Watada H, Imano E, Iwama N, Morishima T, Yamasaki Y, Kajimoto Y, Kamada T: Estrogen regulation of the insulin-like growth factor I gene transcription involves an AP-l enhancer. *J. Biol. Chem.* 269:16433-16442, 1994

[66] Vina J, Sastre J, Pallardo FV, Gambini J, Borras C: Role of mitochondrial oxidative stress to explain the different longevity between genders. Protective effect of estrogens. *Free Radic. Res.* 40:1359-1365, 2006

[67] Walsh BW, Schiff I, Rosner B, Greenberg L, Ravinkar V, Sacks FM: Effects of postmenopausal estrogen replacement on the concentrations and metabolism of plasma lipoproteins. *New England J. Med.* 325:1196-1204, 1991

[68] Wu CT, Chang YL, Shih JY, Lee YC: The significance of estrogen receptor beta in 301 surgically treated non-small cell lung cancers. *J. Thorac Cardiovasc. Surg.* 130:979-986, 2005

Chapter 6

Re-evaluation of the Epidemiological Associations of Female Sexual Steroids and Cancer Risk

Acquittal for the Accused Estrogen

Mild or moderate estrogen deficiency is a relatively frequent, pathologic state of premenopausal women, whereas at menopause ovarian estrogen production definitely declines and serum estrogen levels show further decrease during the postmenopausal life. However, pathologic, excessive estrogen production is extremely rare in women.

Distinction between cancers of moderately and highly estrogen sensitive tumors is necessary, based on their different epidemiological features. Oral cancer is a typical example of the moderately estrogen sensitive tumors and its initiation seems to be associated with a profound estrogen loss [70]. The vast majority of malignancies of the moderately estrogen sensitive organs occur in the late postmenopausal life of women when the ovarian estrogen production is fairly decreased [34].

However, cancers of the highly estrogen sensitive organs such as breast, usually exhibit both premenopausal and postmenopausal occurrence [34,45,66]. In premenopausal cases marked cancer prevalence in organs with high estrogen sensitivity suggests that higher hormone demand of the affected organs results in gene regulation disorders even in mildly or moderately estrogen deficient milieu.

In spite of the different epidemiological data of these two groups of cancers the mechanism of gene regulation disorder in the background of tumor initiation cannot act through quite opposite pathways. Many literary data justify that insulin resistance, obesity and type-2 diabetes are in similarly close association with cancer risk of both highly and moderately estrogen sensitive organs (see Chapter 2). However, the newly revealed association between estrogen deficiency and oral cancer risk means a contradiction of the traditional concept of estrogen induced breast cancer. This contradiction may raise the plausible question, whether increased or decreased serum estrogen levels might be the common risk factors for cancers of highly and moderately estrogen dependent organs?

Risk Factors for Highly Hormone Related Cancers

Cancers of the highly estrogen sensitive organs are in the forefront of tumors as they are regarded as hormone associated ones. They have multicausal origin, however, in the past decades female sexual steroids, especially estrogen was presumed to be an important etiologic factor. The incidence of the so called hormone sensitive tumors such as breast, endometrial and ovarian cancers is highest in the industrialized countries and much lower in the developing countries, with a highest to lowest ratio of 20:1 [2].

Breast tumors are important subjects of cancer research as they are the most frequent cancers in women of the Western world. Marked geographic differences in breast cancer morbidity and mortality seem to be environmental rather than genetic in origin [34]. Migrants from low-incidence to high incidence areas tend to acquire the inclination to cancers characteristic of their adoptive country. Breast cancer risk is significantly higher in North America and northern Europe than in Asia and Africa. As higher economic development is in close correlation with higher prevalence of insulin resistance and obesity, differences in breast cancer incidence may be partially associated with the epidemiological features of metabolic diseases.

The traditional concept of the carcinogenic capacity of the female sex steroid hormones had been based on breast cancer cases [6,32,33,37]. Breast cancer is a tumor of a fairly hormone sensitive tissue, exhibiting both premenopausal and postmenopausal manifestations even without exogenous estrogen treatment [46]. These epidemiological observations can hardly be explained by the carcinogenic capacity of elevated level of female sexual steroids. Moreover, as the majority of malignancies, breast cancer is also a multicausal tumor with strong genetic associations.

Risk factors established or suspected as being associated with breast cancer are numerous [9]. Family history and genetic disposition, lifestyle including diet, physical exercise, smoking, excessive alcohol consumption and individual hormonal and reproductive factors all markedly influence the incidence of this tumor. Recently, insulin resistant states such as obesity, metabolic syndrome and type-2 diabetes are also regarded as strong risk factors for breast cancer (see Chapter 2). Thus hormone replacement therapy (HRT) is only one of a broad range of factors for which an inconsistent association with breast cancer of postmenopausal cases has been found.

Endometrial cancer is the most common invasive malignancy of the female genital tract [27]. The known risk factors associated with an increased risk for endometrial cancer are also numerous. Among others old age, type-2 diabetes, obesity, nulliparity, alcohol use, oral contraception and HRT are regarded as risks for endometrial malignancies [30,74]. However, there are studies, which failed to justify the tumor promoting effect of HRT in the endometrium, even a decreased risk could be observed [3]. Recently, drugs, which have been used for treatment of type-2 diabetes, are important candidates for prevention and possible treatment of endometrial carcinoma [31].

A dualistic model of endometrial carcinogenesis has been proposed earlier [39], which may be important in evaluating the associations of HRT with endometrial cancer. According to this concept, there are two main types of endometrial carcinomas. The first type is a slowly spreading, indolent form, which is supposed to develop in association with excessive estrogen stimulation (type I). The second type is a more aggressive variant considered to arise in a relatively estrogen-deficient milieu of elderly women (type II)! The type I form of endometrial cancer, which may be potentially associated with HRT use, is less aggressive, with a 5-year survival rate of 70-80% [76]. The type II, poorly differentiated endometrial carcinoma affects older women and the 5-year survival rate is shorter, or about 60%.

Recently, a third type of mucinous endometrial carcinoma has been associated with the use of tamoxifen, which is an estrogen antagonist drug used against estrogen receptor positive breast cancers [30,72].

Hyperestrogenism is regarded as a causal factor for endometrial hyperplasia and later to epithelial atypia, which may be the predecessor of endometrial adenocarcinoma [14]. However, hormone treatment of postmenopausal women should not be considered extreme but rather an endeavor to achieve a physiological estrogen level. Approximately 2-3% of the women under continuous combined HRT show proliferative endometrial activity, but almost all without any signs of atypical hyperplasia [30,47,64].

An important parallelism between breast and endometrial cancers is that only the estrogen receptor positive, highly differentiated, slow growing forms have been assumed to have associations with HRT use [18,30].

Ovarian cancer represents about 30% of all malignancies of the female genital tract. The age adjusted incidence rates vary from <2/100 000 women in most of Southest Asia and Africa to >15/100 000 cases in Northern and Eastern Europe [2]. The economically advanced countries of North America and Europe show the highest rates.

The incidence of ovarian cancer shows a steady increase with age. Reduced risk of the disease is consistently associated with high parity and oral contraceptive use [76]. Energy rich diet and insulin resistance have also been related to ovarian cancer [8]. Literary data suggest that treatments used against insulin resistance emerge as effective tools in prevention and cure of endometrial cancers [31].

Associations between HRT and ovarian cancer are fairly controversial. A review of 20 studies on ovarian cancer reached no satisfactory conclusion concerning HRT risk for this tumor [52]. Five studies described a slightly elevated ovarian cancer risk in HRT users [25,35,48,58,75], whereas the other 15 studies did not. Recently, further doubts concerning associations between HRT use and ovarian cancer risk have emerged [62].

Shortcomings of Studies on Correlations of HRT Use and Cancer Risk

The postmenopausal period in women is a physiological model for studies on the hormonal, metabolic and gene regulation changes associated with estrogen deficiency. In healthy postmenopausal women there are physiological mechanisms to adapt to the gradual loss of estrogen signals. However, this new equilibrium comprises many risks and traps for slipping out of the regular metabolic and hormonal pathways.

An abrupt decrease in estrogen hormone levels either after a natural or an artificial menopause may cause gene regulation disturbances not only in the female reproductive system but also in many other organs. Radical or subtotal hysterectomy in premenopausal women results in a sudden, definite loss of ovarian estrogen synthesis and may cause severe consequences, especially without HRT use. Spontaneous or induced abortion also causes a transitory but shocking fall in the hormone levels.

In clinical practice about 40% of women have severe menopausal complaints, which usually require medical help [26]. Menopausal complaints are not only unpleasant, bothering symptoms but suggest thorough disorders of adaptation to estrogen loss and a possibility for altered gene regulation. The alterations may affect the general health of the women, as they are risks for both cardiovascular diseases and malignancies. If estrogen deficiency is regarded as a risk for cancers these patients have a greater cancer risk in their later life as compared with women who have gradually, asymptomatically lost their estrogen signals and have no need for HRT use. These considerations suggest that cancer risk in aged women, among other factors, may depend on their endogenous hormonal characteristics, their menopausal process and on HRT use in their history.

Correct evaluation of correlations between HRT use and cancer risk requires strict selection of the patients included, proper length of the observational period and awareness of estrogen receptor positivity of tumors.

Selection of Patients for HRT Studies

Cancers are multicausal diseases, and the carcinogenic capacity of the physiological levels of female sexual steroids is hardly, if at all justifiable. Investigation of HRT use, as a supposed cancer risk factor on pooled, unselected population of women is misleading.

Supposedly, neither the hormone treated nor the untreated groups of women involved in the HRT studies are homogenous. The marked differences in menopausal processes in women and their various effects on gene regulation may partially explain the controversies concerning the associations of HRT and cancer.

Correlations between HRT use and breast cancer risk are usually examined in two groups of involved women; with and without hormone treatment, disregarding their individual hormonal and reproductive differences and other known or suspected risk factors. In these studies the majority of HRT user women may be assumed to have severe postmenopausal complaints in connection with a failure of the adaptation mechanisms. However, women without hormone treatment may have predominantly uneventful perimenopausal period due to their good adaptation. Consequently, the epidemiological studies on breast cancer risk of HRT users reflect an additive effect of the endogenous hormonal features of the HRT user population and of their hormone treatment.

A collaborative re-analysis was performed on data from 51 epidemiological studies dealing mainly with single estrogen substitution [15]. The overall relative risk for breast cancer was as low as 1.14 when HRT users were compared with never users. The increase in the risk was small but significant because of the great number of examined cases [18]. However, a WHI publication could find no risk for breast cancer among women who used estrogen alone, even unopposed estrogen treatment was associated with a possible reduction in breast cancer risk (HR: 0.77) [5]. The WHI authors suggested that this reduction in breast cancer risk associated to HRT requires further investigation. This valuable study seems to be a stretching force against the old frame of carcinogenicity of estrogen.

The small differences in breast cancer risk between HRT user and untreated populations of women - even advantageously decreased breast cancer risk as a result of one-armed estrogen treatment - raise the possibility of bias and improper patient selection in the majority of studies [18].

How can we explain the results of the widespread epidemiological studies, which support the slightly but consequently higher breast cancer risk in postmenopausal women with HRT use as compared with untreated cases?

Estrogen deficiency seems to be a cancer risk factor, especially for highly estrogen sensitive organs. Women belonging to the group of HRT users supposedly have severe postmenopausal complaints based on failure of their adaptation. Consequently, HRT users have a higher risk for breast cancer initiation as compared with complaint-free women without treatment.

Presumably, the beneficial effect of HRT use may decrease the rate of new cancer initiation in postmenopausal women. However, the pre-existing subclinical cancers induced by the pre- or perimenopausal hormonal disorders cannot be completely destroyed. Consequently, an elevated breast cancer incidence may remain in the group of endangered women with severe endogenous hormone deficiency and/or defective adaptation mechanism in spite of HRT use. These considerations may explain the slightly but consequently elevated breast cancer risk among HRT users as compared with untreated women with physiological adaptation.

Furthermore, the estrogen deficiency theory justifies that in a methodologically stronger WHI study an unexpected, beneficial effect of HRT use against breast cancer was observed [5]. One-armed HRT was applied on 10 793 women with prior hysterectomy by conjugated estrogen and it was found to be associated with reduction of breast cancer risk. This result justifies the importance of selection of homogenously endangered patients for epidemiological studies and supports the protective role of estrogen against breast cancer.

The effects of adaptation disorders on breast cancer risk should be prospectively studied via comparison of untreated patients with and without postmenopausal complaints. Moreover, associations of HRT use and breast cancer risk might be correctly examined if the cases and controls have similar menopausal histories.

Dynamics of Cancer Growth and Length of the Observational Period

Dynamics of breast cancer initiation and promotion is still poorly understood [1,9,29,40,50,77]. Thus, firm causal conclusions cannot be established from the associations between hormone treatment and breast cancer found on inhomogeneous female populations.

Studies on HRT user women failed to clarify whether hormone treatment apparently stimulates induction of cancers de novo by initiating mutations, or facilitates the growth of pre-existing, small tumors [18].

The tumor doubling time (TDT) concept is useful for assessment of the duration of prediagnostic stage of cancers. It is defined as the time for a tumor volume or cell number to double once [68]. TDT depends on many variables such as rate of cell division, proportion of actively dividing cells, rate of apoptoses, angiogenetic potential, intermitotic interval, shedding of tumor cells, ratio of tumor and stromal cells and so on. These numerous factors explain the wide range of estimations of TDT in breast cancer [63,67]. Current data show that a median TDT for human cancers may be 50-100 days [68].

A size of 1 cm in diameter is more or less the smallest tumor to be diagnosed clinically. This corresponds to rough and ready 10^9 cells but this number depends strongly on the tumor cell size [67]. This means that on average at least 1750-3500 days (5-10 years) are necessary from the initial mutation to a clinically and/or mammographically detectable tumor mass [28]. However, this calculation is true for a tumor only in case of ideal circumstances and does not consider the cell loss by apoptosis, death and shedding [68]. Further, there are no data concerning the time demand of the transition from an intraepithelial, non-invasive cancer to an invasive one, which will further prolong the period from tumor initiation to clinical cancer diagnosis [18]. In reality, the estimated time from initiation to a diagnosable cancer might be much longer than 5-10 years.

Considering the theories on tumor growth dynamics, the presumable time between supposed initiation of breast tumors by HRT and clinical detection seems to be at least 10 years or even longer [18]. All the studies showing associations between HRT and breast cancer are based on far shorter observational periods.

Awareness of Estrogen Receptor Positivity of Cancers

The mechanisms of initiation versus promotion of hormone sensitive cancers, particularly breast cancer, are only scarcely understood. A widespread theory is that hormonal influence of breast cancer is necessary from the primordial mutation to clinical cancer diagnosis after many years [4,17].

The pathophysiological prerequisite for the initiation and progression of hormone induced cancer in postmenopausal women and its association with HRT use is the presence of active estrogen receptors in the target tissues [18]. However, it is a well-known fact that estrogen receptor expression is fairly different in breast cancers and there are also receptor-negative tumors. Unfortunately, the studies, which formed the current view on the HRT-induced cancer risk did not incorporate biochemical or immunohistochemical data to clarify levels of estrogen receptor expression of breast cancers [18]. These shortcomings may also explain the controversial associations of HRT and breast cancer risk and the results become questionable.

Doubts concerning HRT induced cancer initiation. Majority of breast cancers detected in association with HRT use are histologically well differentiated and have a relatively good prognosis [18]. These are usually slowly growing cancers and do not metastasize early. Generally, the low-grade breast cancers with low malignancy are estrogen receptor positive. As hormone receptors are the prerequisites for the theoretical impact of HRT use on breast cancer initiation, only the differentiated, receptor positive cancers with slow progression may be associated with hormonal influences.

However, initiation of both ER-positive and ER-negative breast cancers may be equally possible based on the estrogen deficiency theory. Gene regulation disturbance caused by estrogen loss does not require normal ER signals, in contrast, overwhelming growth factor activities become predominant versus non-liganded, altered ERs. By this way estrogen deficiency may induce either highly differentiated, receptor-positive or poorly differentiated receptor-negative cancers.

ER-positive breast cancers are predominantly slow growing tumors requiring longer period between presumed HRT-induced initiation and clinical cancer diagnosis as compared with undifferentiated, receptor negative ones. Consequently, for hormone receptor positive, highly differentiated cancers an even much longer observational period would be necessary to establish the correlation between HRT use and breast cancer risk.

In contrast, estrogen deficiency induced breast cancer may be initiated in the pre- or perimenopausal period by moderate estrogen loss previous to the beginning of HRT. At menopause a further, abrupt decrease of estrogen level may provoke postmenopausal complaints and at the same time, faster growth of the pre-existing cancer. However, HRT use will alleviate the complaints and diminish the aggressivity of the early cancer. This explanation illuminates both the possibility of clinical cancer diagnosis after 4-5 years of HRT use and the lower aggressivity of cancers associated with hormone treatment.

Doubts concerning HRT induced cancer promotion. Dietel et al. proposed that as the observation time of women with HRT use is not long enough, hormones may not initiate but perhaps may accelerate the tumor growth leading to an earlier clinical discovery. A contradictory result with HRT associated promotion of breast cancer is the slower growth, reduced aggressivity of tumors and longer survival among HRT user women as compared with those who did not take HRT [18]. Nevertheless, as only hormone sensitive tumors may be affected by HRT and hormone receptor expression means a higher differentiation of breast cancers, it is not probable that hormone treatment induces dedifferentiation and more rapid progression of tumors.

Cancer initiation and promotion are generally not contradictory processes. There are many factors, including hormonal signals, which may induce both cancer initiation and promotion. Increased rates of tumor initiation and progression have been observed in compensatory hyperinsulinemia associated with insulin resistance. Elevated insulin and concomitantly elevated IGF levels are proven risk factors for both breast cancer initiation and progression (see Chapter 2). In case of another hormone, such as estrogen, an inverse effect on tumor initiation as compared to tumor promotion is hardly justifiable.

Anticancer Capacity of HRT Use in Several Organs

Decisive proofs against HRT-induced cancer initiation are the recently published beneficial anticancer effects of hormone treatment against moderately and highly hormone dependent tumors at several sites. Favorable effects of HRT use have been published in relation to oral, esophageal, gastric, colorectal, lung, cervical, liver and urinary bladder cancers [13,21,22,24,36,51,52,58]. Recently, similar protective effect of HRT has been observed against the highly estrogen sensitive breast and endometrial cancers [3,5]. Explanation to these widespread epidemiological data is quite impossible based on the theory of estrogen-induced carcinogenesis.

Recently, there have been studies on the different activities of estrogen and ERs on various cell groups (see Chapter 5). However, the carcinogenic and anticancer capacity of such an important hormone may not be reconciled even on cells with fairly different structure and function.

Estrogen Deficiency and Cancer Risk in Postmenopausal Women

Cancer development requires many years from initiation to clinical appearance, and this is valid also for estrogen deficient postmenopausal women, especially if the main exogenous cancer risk factors are missing (see Chapter 8). The majority of postmenopausal cancers may be initiated at the perimenopausal or postmenopausal estrogen deficient period and the clinical manifestation occurs much later. As the average age at menopause is about 50 years in Hungary, the age above 60 may be especially dangerous for clinical appearance of malignancies at moderately estrogen sensitive sites in women.

Smoking associated tumors can be regarded as typically *moderately estrogen sensitive malignancies* such as cancers of the oral cavity, pharynx, larynx, lung and urinary bladder. Their incidence exhibits very high male to female ratios and has controversial correlations with HRT use. Recent literary data support that postmenopausal hormone therapy seems to have advantageous anticancer impact on these types of cancers (see Chapter 4). These observations suggest that estrogen loss in postmenopausal women may have crucial role in development of smoking-related cancers, which seems to be independent of smoking habits [59,70].

Oral cancer is a typically smoking-associated tumor with high male to female ratio and is regarded as moderately hormone sensitive type. Almost exclusively *postmenopausal state* of the female oral cancer patients suggested that estrogen deficiency has crucial role in the development of this tumor. The length of interval between their menopause and tumor onset proved also to be decisive factor in the clinical appearance of oral cancer. Fairly long mean interval between menopause of oral cancer cases and tumor diagnosis (near 17 years) suggested an important role of estrogen deprivation in oral cancer initiation [70,71]. The longer the postmenopausal period of estrogen deficiency the higher the possibility of clinical manifestation of tumors initiated by estrogen loss.

An early menopause, such as premature ovarian failure under 40 years or premenopausal hysterectomy with or without ovarectomy mean a *shorter hormonally active reproductive period* and may have thorough consequences affecting gene regulation. A significantly higher ratio of young age (<45 yrs) at menopause among the female oral cancer cases as compared with the age-matched tumor-free controls was demonstrated.

Moreover, a *sudden loss of the estrogen signal* may be an especially dangerous shock for the regulatory mechanisms both in the highly and moderately estrogen sensitive organs. Hysterectomy with or without ovarectomy proved to be a high risk factor for oral cancer among women in our epidemiological study.

Cancers of the highly estrogen sensitive organs such as breast cancer may also occur in older postmenopausal cases. In these women a good hormonal equilibrium may be presumed during their reproductive period, which defends the highly hormone sensitive organs from cancer initiation. The first shock of estrogen loss arises in the perimenopausal period, which may serve as cancer initiator. However, the continuously decreasing ovarian estrogen synthesis during postmenopausal life may be a sword of Damocles for all organs.

Moderate Estrogen Deficiency and Cancer Risk in Premenopausal Women

The carcinogenic effects of marked estrogen deficiency may easily be studied in women, since their life is clearly separated into premenopausal and postmenopausal periods. However, the long-term systemic effects of mildly or moderately decreased estrogen levels in premenopausal women maybe hardly clarified.

In premenopausal women there are many pathological states predisposing to mild or moderate estrogen deficiency. Ovarian insufficiency may result in long or irregular menstrual cycles and unexplained infertility. Chronic anovulation and ovulatory dysfunction were found also to be associated with increased prevalence of endometrial cancer [16,66]. Spontaneous and induced abortions provoke sudden decrease of the highly elevated estrogen level and may be regarded as transitory periods with increased inclination to disorders of gene regulation. Literary data are controversial concerning the associations of abortion and breast cancer risk; however, late termination of pregnancy at abortion seems to be a high risk for breast cancer (see Chapter 4).

Immunosuppressive therapy against autoimmune diseases, cancer or rejection reaction in organ transplantation cases may also induce ovarian insufficiency and risk for development of malignancies.

Polycystic ovarian syndrome (PCOS) is a complex disorder that is presumably caused by a large number of different genetic abnormalities. PCOS is the most common endocrinopathy of women in reproductive age [23,54,61]. PCOS seems to be a pathological model of hormonal and metabolic alterations of postmenopausal status in premenopausal women. It may usually be manifested by menstrual disorders, anovulation, infertility, hirsutism and obesity and means a conspicuously increased risk for cancers at highly estrogen sensitive sites [23,54,69].

Some authors suppose that unopposed estrogen levels continuously stimulate ERs in women with PCOS, which maybe a risk for endometrial and breast cancers [23]. However, insulin resistance and hyperinsulinemia in patients with PCOS are associated with high ovarian androgen synthesis and estrogen deficiency [49].

Infertility is the most sensitive indicator of hormonal disorders in symptom-free women. PCOS cases diagnosed among adolescents suggest that the disease may develop insidiously during puberty rather than at a later time of presentation of infertility [61]. Consequently, the hormonal insufficiency may be long lasting enough to promote cancer development in young adulthood of affected women.

PCOS has a great significance as latent, undiagnosed cases are relatively numerous among the female population [12,56]. If the diagnosis is based on the morphological findings of ovarian pathology at either surgery or ultrasonography, then up to 20% of unselected women have been reported to be affected [19,56]. Or about 25% of these women have no clinical symptoms although many do have laboratory findings suggesting endocrinologic and metabolic disturbances associated with PCOS such as hyperandrogenism and hyperinsulinemia [7].

As PCOS-associated endocrine alterations mean risk factors for breast and gynecological cancers. In otherwise healthy, young premenopausal patients with unexpected malignancies a thorough endocrinologic examination should be performed.

Bewildering Differences between Cancer Epidemiology of Highly and Moderately Estrogen Sensitive Organs

Epidemiological studies on the incidence rate of moderately estrogen sensitive cancers provide the possibility to compare the data of the two genders, whereas in case of highly hormone sensitive cancers of women this advantage is excluded.

The most important source of misunderstandings and misinterpretations in the epidemiology of highly estrogen sensitive breast cancer may be that its exhibition is almost exclusively restricted to one gender. On the contrary, in case of the moderately hormone sensitive oral cancer, gender-related epidemiological differences and their trends have raised many questions to be answered (see Chapter 1). Moreover, the gender-related differences in oral cancer epidemiology served as leaders on the route from smoking associated cancers to the discovery of estrogen deficiency induced carcinogenesis.

Recently estrogen and its receptors are regarded as pivotal gene regulators affecting cell growth, proliferation, differentiation and metabolism (see Chapter 5). Cells of all tissues and organs have estrogen receptors with variable expression levels and they are deeply influenced by estrogen receptor signal induced mechanisms even out of the female genital tract. Therefore, assumption of a strict distinction or even inverse mechanisms between carcinogenesis in highly and moderately estrogen sensitive organs is not reasonable.

Cancers of the *highly estrogen sensitive breast, endometrium and ovary* have some special characteristics even without exogenous hormone treatment. They have no sharp distinction concerning the incidence rate between premenopausal and postmenopausal cases.

Epidemiological data on cancers of the highly estrogen sensitive organs show a relatively wide range of ages among patients. Moreover, among breast cancer cases at least 25-30% of the affected women are premenopausal [34]. Recently, in a prospective study on breast cancer cases even more than 50% of the patients were premenopausal [46]. These data suggest that for the highly estrogen sensitive organs even a mild or moderate estrogen deficiency in young, premenopausal cases is enough to initiate gene regulation disorders.

Breast cancer, which is a typical example of cancers of the highly hormone related tissues, is quite uncommon in women younger than 30 years of age. Thereafter, the breast cancer risk steadily increases throughout the life and after menopause the upward slope of the curve is much less steep [34]. Endometrial cancer may also occur in young women and up to 30% of the cases may be premenopausal [66].

These epidemiological data seem to support the carcinogenic capacity of moderate estrogen deficiency in young, premenopausal cases affecting both tumor initiation and promotion. Development of decreased or instable estrogen levels may be originated in adolescence and it may be completely symptom-free apart from the fertility problems. Organs with high estrogen demand may be disturbed in their gene regulation at very young ages by hormonal disorders. Insidious, mild estrogen deficiency may result in development of diagnosable breast, endometrial or ovarian tumor in young adults.

Later, the disorders of the hormonal equilibrium show a continuously increasing prevalence with age. Transitory or definite estrogen loss in the reproductive period caused by endogenous ovarian insufficiency, abortions, therapeutic measures or other causes may result in increasing prevalence of cancers in the highly hormone sensitive organs.

Among premenopausal PCOS cases with hormonal disorders an increased prevalence of cancers could be observed preferentially in the breast, endometrium and ovary [54,55,61,69]. In a mortality study on patients with PCOS breast cancer proved to be the leading cause of death [54].

In the postmenopausal life further increase of breast cancer incidence can be observed. Initiation of breast tumors diagnosed in cases within 1-5 years after menopause may not be associated with either the exact date of the last menstruation or with HRT use. Tumor induction in these cases may be originated from a long lasting pre- or perimenopausal hormonal deficiency. Moreover, the postmenopausal abrupt decrease of estrogen levels may help the faster growth of a pre-existing, subclinical cancer.

Cancers of the *moderately estrogen sensitive organs* occur typically in older cases among women [34] and they are supposedly postmenopausal suggestive of a profound estrogen loss in association with initiation of these tumors. Moderately estrogen sensitive cancers show striking differences in prevalence and age related distribution in the two genders.

The male to female ratios of oral cancer showed a conspicuous dromedary-shape curve when they were studied in different age groups (Figure 6.1). Shockingly young oral cancer cases less than 30 years of age are extremely rare. Among them the effect of traditional, exogenous risk factors such as excessive alcohol intake or tobacco may be excluded, and a low male to female ratio or even predominance of female cases could be observed (see Chapter 1).

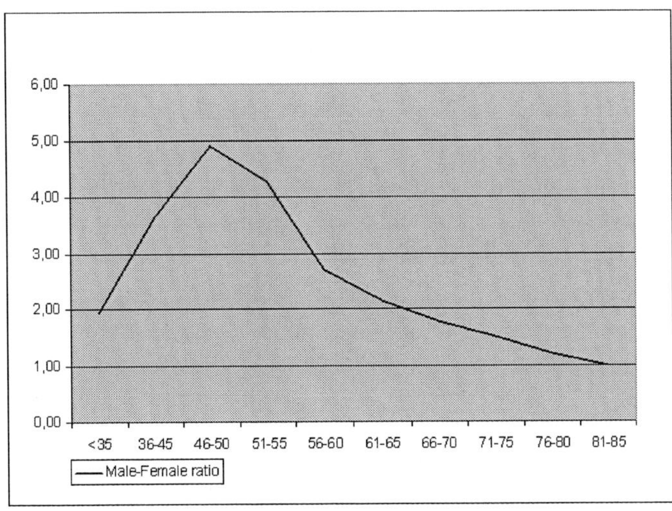

Figure 6.1. Male to female ratio of oral cancer patients depending on their age shows a dromedary like curve and a steep decline begins at 51-55 years of age.

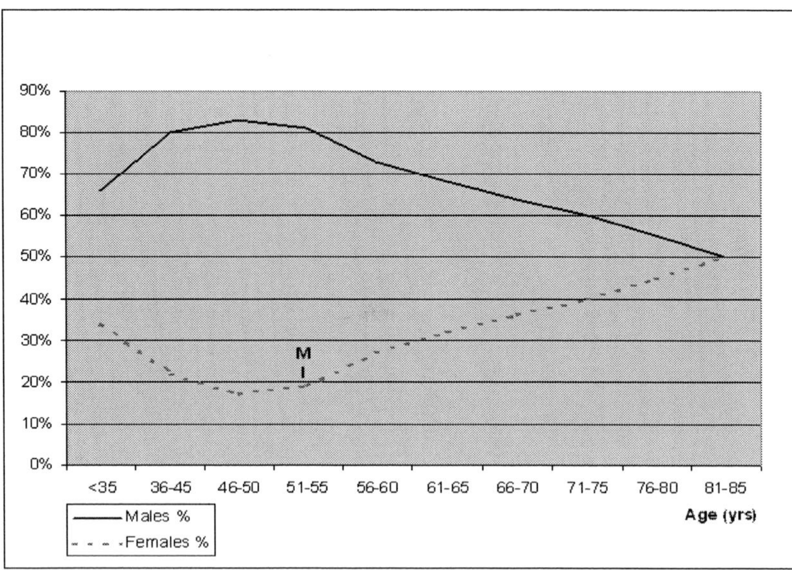

Figure 6.2. Percentage of male and female cases among oral cancer patients depending on their age. Between 40 and 60 years of age the male to female ratio is constantly high. At mean age of menopause (M) an increasing trend of cancer incidence among females but a decreasing trend among males can be observed.

In young women oral cancer initiation requires more profound estrogen deficiency from their adolescence as compared with the highly estrogen sensitive cancers. As oral cancer has a multicausal origin, a further possibility is the coexistence of mild estrogen deficiency with other non-traditional cancer risk factors. Similar, estrogen deficient states are probably extremely rare in young boys; theoretically rather androgen excess may provoke their gene regulation disorders. These differences in hormonal disorders may explain the equalization of the male to female ratio of oral cancer among cases less than 30 years of age.

Oral cancer incidence in adult and middle aged female cases (between 40-60 yrs) is rare as healthy women in their reproductive period enjoy the protective effect of female sexual steroids against cancers. Moreover, moderately estrogen sensitive cancers are rarely associated with mild hormonal disorders. Consequently, oral cancer cases between the ages of 40 and 60 exhibit the highest male to female ratio because of the low incidence rate of women. As clinical cancer diagnosis from perimenopausal tumor initiation requires at least 10 years or more, the male to female ratio of diagnosable oral cancer remains high till the age of early 60s.

However, above the age of 60, or about 10 years after the mean age at menopause a steeply increasing ratio of female oral cancer cases as compared with males justifies the tumor inductive effect of a sudden estrogen decrease at menopause. Percentage of male and female cases among oral cancer patients depending on their age exhibits characteristic curves (Figure 6.2). These age-dependent, gender related differences in oral cancer prevalence might plausibly derive from the coarse hormonal changes between the reproductive and postmenopausal periods of women.

Extraovarian Estrogen Synthesis

There are recently clarified possibilities for extraovarian estrogen synthesis in postmenopausal women. In premenopausal women and estrous animals, the principal source of estradiol is ovarian, however, during reproductive senescence a significant amount of estradiol is produced extragonadally.

Female sexual steroids may be synthesized from precursor steroids by aromatase enzyme activity in many cell and tissue types included vascular endothelium, bone, brain, breast and endometrium [41,42,45,60,73]. Surprisingly, these are the very tissues evidently endangered by an estrogen deficient milieu and the severe consequences are cardiovascular disease, osteoporosis and ischemic injuries of the central nervous system. Similarly, aromatase activity and extragonadal estrogen synthesis in the highly estrogen sensitive breast and endometrium suggest important defensive roles in postmenopausal women against cancer initiation.

Some authors regarded estrogen accumulation in the breast tissue of postmenopausal women as justification of hormone induced carcinogenesis in estrogen deficient cases (see Chapter 4). However, it is not probable that a biological process serves as facilitation of cancer development. Rather, it may be a defensive mechanism, as highly estrogen sensitive tissues have increased inclination to cancer initiation in a hormone deficient milieu.

Risk of Antiestrogen Therapy for Postmenopausal Women with ER-positive Breast Cancer

Estrogen is not simply a regulator of mitogenic activity but has surveillance upon metabolic processes and oxidation equilibrium (Chapters 4, 5 and 7). Antiestrogen treatment has severe side effects, however its therapeutic gain is also questionable.

Antiestrogen treatment of ER-positive breast cancers is an everyday adjuvant therapy. The most important mechanisms of these agents are competitive antagonism on estrogen receptors or inhibition of aromatase enzyme to block estrogen synthesis. Adjuvant therapy with the estrogen antagonist tamoxifen was considered the gold-standard treatment against ER-positive breast cancers.

Tamoxifen use was associated with elevated risks of endometrial cancer incidence and mortality and uterine sarcomas seemed also to be overrepresented among women using tamoxifen. [38]. Aromatase inhibitors had substantial benefit in terms of tolerability of side effects; however, accelerated bone resorption was exhibited in treated postmenopausal women [10].

Astroglial aromatase activity and extragonadal estrogen production in the brain is a key to endogenous neuroprotection in female cases. Aromatase inhibitor treatment in postmenopausal women could have detrimental impact on ischemic brain [41].

Tamoxifen is a powerful inhibitor of the mitochondrial electron transport chain. It causes significant rise in mitochondrial lipid peroxidation, protein carbonyl content and superoxide radical generation. Taurine treatment was suggested to ameliorate tamoxifen-induced mitochondrial toxicity and to increase free radical-scavenging activity [53].

The ineffective or insufficient anticancer capacity of estrogen inhibitors in breast cancer cases was regarded as "resistance" against the therapy. Nowadays, there are plenty of experimental data on cross talks and interplays between receptors of estrogen and growth factors (Chapter 5). Some researchers correctly assumed that inhibition of estrogen effect may provoke overwhelming predominance of growth factors, which leads to failure of tumor therapy. However, they tried to solve this contradiction by parallel inhibition of both estrogen and growth factor receptors [43,44].

Unfortunately, the principle of tumor treatment by antiestrogen compounds is completely deceptive. Ineffectivity and harmful side effects of these "drugs" may be eliminated by complete abandonment of their use.

Estrogen Deficiency in Men

In men, the metabolic importance of the estrogen milieu has been newly recognized, and today its role in male physiology seems to be also essential [20].

Complete estrogen deficiency in males is extremely rare such as aromatase deficiency and estrogen resistance [11,65]. Examinations on these sporadic male cases resulted in striking findings concerning metabolic disorders, such as severe type-2 diabetes being resistant to usual therapy. In these totally estrogen deficient males type-2 diabetes may be treated by estrogen administration. Of course, these sporadic estrogen deficient male cases cannot supply any information concerning the long-term effects, even the carcinogenicity of their hormonal disorder.

Currently, the pathophysiological effects of moderate estrogen deficiency in men and its consequences are quite obscure. Based on the findings found in female cases, disturbed equilibrium of sexual steroids and especially estrogen deficiency may also be important cancer risk factors in men. This will probably be a more difficult though exiting area for further investigations.

References

[1] Adami HO, Signorello LB, and Trichopolos D: Towards an understanding of breast cancer etiology. *Semin. Cancer Biol.* 8:255-262, 1998

[2] American Institute For Cancer Research /World cancer Research Fund Food, nutrition and the prevention of cancer: a global perspective. American Institute of Cancer Research, Washington, DC, 252-287, 2002

[3] Anderos GL, Judd HL, Kaunitz AM et al: Womens's Health Intitative Investigator Effects of estrogen plus progestin on gynaecologic cancers and associated diagnostic producers: The Women's Health Intitative randomised trial. *JAMA* 290:1739-1748, 2003

[4] Anderson TJ, Battersby S, King RJB et al: Oral contraceptive use influences resting breast proliferation. *Hum. Pathol.* 20:1139-1144, 1989

[5] Anderson GL, Limacher M, Assaf AR, Bassford T, Beresford SA, Black H, Bonds D, Brunner R, Brzyski R, Caan B, Chlebowski R, Curb D, Gass M, Hays J, Heiss G, Hendrix S, Howard BV, Hsia J, Hubbell A, Jackson R, Johnson KC, Judd H, Kotchen JM, Kuller L, LaCroix AZ, Lane D, Langer RD, Lasser N, Lewis CE, Manson J, Margolis K, Ockene J, O'Sullian MJ, Phillips L, Prentice RL, Ritenbaugh C, Robbins J, Rossouw JE, Sarto G, Stefanick ML, Van Horn L, Wactawski-Wende J, Wallace R, Wassertheil-Smoller S: Women's Health Intitative Steering Committee. Effects of conjugated equine estrogen in postmenopausal women with hysterctomy: the Women's Health Intitative randomized controlled trial. *JAMA* 291:1701-1712, 2004

[6] Berrino F, Muti P, Micheli A, Bolelli G, Krogh V, Sciajno R et al: Serum sex hormon levels after menopause and subsequent breast cancer. *J. Natl. Cancer Inst.* 88:291-296, 1996

[7] Bloomgarden ZT: Second World Congress on the Insulin Resistance Syndrome: Mediators, pediatric insulin resistance, the polycystic ovary syndrome, and malignancy. *Diabetes Care* 28:1821-1830, 2005

[8] Bosetti C, Negri E, Franceschi S, Pelucchi C, Talamini R, Montella M, Conti E, La Vecchia C: Diet and ovarian cancer risk: a case-control study in Italy. *Int. J. Cancer* 93:911-915, 2001

[9] Brekelmans CT: Risk factors and risk reduction of breast and ovarian cancer. *Curr. Opin. Obstet Gynecol.* 15:63-68, 2003

[10] Buzdar AU, Coombes RC, Goss PE, Winer EP: Summary of aromatase inhibitor clinical trials in postmenopausal women with early breast cancer. *Cancer* 112 (3 Suppl):700-709, 2008

[11] Carani C, Qin K, Simoni M, Faustini-Fustini M, Serpente S, Boyd J et al: Effect of testosterone and estradiol a in man with aromatase deficiency. *New Engl. J. Med.* 337:91-95, 1997

[12] Carmina E, Lobo RA: Polycystic ovaries in hirsute women with normal menses. *Am. J. Med.* 111:602-606, 2001

[13] Castelao JE, Yuan J-M, Skipper PL, Tannenbaum SR, Gago-Dominguez M, Crowder JS, Ross RK, Yu MC: Gender and smoking-related bladder cancer risk. *J. Natl. Cancer Inst.* 93:538-545, 2001

[14] Cirisano FD, Robboy SJ, Dodge RK, Bentley RC, Krigman HR, Synan IS, Soper JT, Clarke Pearson DL: The outcome of state I-II clinically and surgically staged papillary serous and clear cell endometrial cancers when compared with endometrial carcinoma. *Gynecol. Oncol.* 77:55-65, 2000

[15] Collaborative Group on Hormonal Factors in Breast Cancer: Collaborative reanalysis of data from 51 epidemiological studies of 52 705 women with breast cancer and 108 411 women without breast cancer. *Lancet* 350:1047-1059, 1997

[16] Coulam CB, Annegers JF, Kranz JS: Chronic anovulation syndrome and associated neoplasia. *Obstet Gynecol.* 61:403-407, 1983

[17] Cutuli B, Dhermain F, Magrini SM, Wasserman TH, Bogart JA et al: Breast cancer occurred after treatment for Hodgkin's disease: analysis of 133 cases. *Radiother. Oncol.* 59:247-255, 2001

[18] Dietel M, Lewis MA, Shapiro S: Hormone replacement therapy: pathobiological aspects of hormone-sensitive cancers in women relevant to epidemiological studies on HRT: a mini-review. *Human Reprod.* 20:2052-2060, 2005

[19] Farquhar CM, Birdsall M, Manning P et al: The prevalence of polycystic ovaries on ultrasound scanning in a population of randomly selected women. *Aust. NZ Obstet Gynaecol.* 34:67-72, 1994

[20] Faustini-Fustini M, Rochira V, Carani C: Oestrogen deficiency in men: where are we today? *Eur. J. Endocrinol.* 140:111-129, 1999

[21] Fernandez E, La Vecchia C, Balducci A, Chatenoud L, Franceschi S, Negri E: Oral contraceptives and colorectal cancer risk: a meta-analysis. *Br. J. Cancer* 84:722-727, 2001

[22] Fernandez E, Gallus S, Bosetti C, Franceschi S, Negri E, La Vecchia C: Hormone replacement therapy and cancer risk: a systematic analysis from a network of case-control studies. *Int. J. Cancer* 105:408-412, 2003

[23] Gadducci A, Gargini A, Palla E, Fanucchi A, Genazzani AR: Polycystic ovary syndrome and gynecological cancers: is there a link? *Gynecol. Endocrinol.* 20:200-208, 2005

[24] Gallus S, Bosetti C, Franceschi S, Levi F, Simonato L, Negri E, La Vecchia C: Oesophageal cancer in women: tobacco, alcohol, nutritional and hormonal factors. *Br. J. Cancer* 85:341-345, 2001

[25] Gambacciani M, Rosano GM, Monteleone P, Fini M and Genazziani AR: Clinical relevance of the HERS trial. *Lancet* 360:641, 2002

[26] Grady D: Postmenopausal hormones – therapy for symptoms only. *New Engl. J. Med.* 348:1-3, 2003

[27] Greenle RT, Murray T, Bolden S, Wongo PA: Cancer statistics. CA *Cancer J. Clin.* 50:7-33, 2000

[28] Haskell CM: Thorax. Unknown primary-breast cancer in cancer treatment, 2nd ed. WB Saunders Company 1985

[29] Hofseth LJ, Raafat AM, Osuch JR, Pathak DR, Slomski CA, Haslam SZ: Hormone replacement therapy with estrogen or estrogen plus medroxy-progesterone acetate is associated with increased epithelial proliferation in the normal postmenopausal breast. *J. Clin. Endocrinol. Metab.* 84:4559-4565, 1999

[30] Horn LC, Dietel M, Einenkel J: Hormone replacement therapy (HRT) and endometrial morphology under consideration of the different molecular pathways in endometrial carcinogenesis. *Eur. J. Obst. Gyn. Repr. Biol.* 122:4-12, 2005

[31] Ito K, Utsunomiya H, Yaegashi N, Sasano H: Biological roles of estrogen and progesterone in human endometrial carcinoma – new developments in potential endocrine therapy for endometrial cancer. *Endocrine Journal* 54:667-679, 2007

[32] Kabuto M, Akiba S, Stevens RG, Neriishi K, Land CE: A prospective study of estradiol and breast cancer in Japanese women. *Cancer Epidemiol. Biomark and Prev.* 9:575-579, 2000

[33] Key TJ, Applyby PN, Reeves GK: Body mass index, serum sex hormones and breast cancer risk in postmenopausal women. *J. Natl. Cancer Inst.* 95:1218-1226, 2003

[34] Kumar V, Abbas AK, Fausto N, Mitchell RN: Robbins Basic Pathology. 8th edition Saunders Elsevier 2007

[35] Lacey JV, Mink PJ, Lubin JH, Sherman ME, Troisi R, Hartge P, Schatzkin A, Schairer C: Menopausal hormone replacement therapy and risk of ovarian cancer. *J. Am. Med.* Assoc 288:334-341, 2002

[36] La Vecchia C, D'Avanzo B, Franceschi S, Negri E, Parazzini F, Decarli A: Menstrual and reproductive factors and gastric-cancer risk in women. *Int. J. Cancer* 59:761-764, 1994

[37] La Vecchia C, Brinton LA, McTiernan A: Menopause, hormone replacement therapy and cancer. *Maturitas* 39:97-115, 2001

[38] Lavie O, Barnett-Grines O, Narod SA, Rennert G: The risk of developing uterine sarcoma after tamoxifen use. *Int. J. Gynec. Cancer* 18:352-356, 2008

[39] Lax SF, Kendall B, Tashiro H, Slebos RJC, Hedrick L: Analysis of p53 and K-ras mutations and microsatellite instability suggests distinct molecular genetic pathways in the pathogenesis of uterine endometrioid and serous carcinoma. *Cancer* 88:814-824, 2000

[40] Li CI, Weiss NS, Stanford JL, Daling JR: Hormone replacement therapy in relation to risk of lobular and ductal breast carcinoma in middle-aged women. *Cancer* 88:2570-2577, 2000

[41] McCullough LD, Blizzard K, Simpson ER, Öz OK, Hurn PD: Aromatase cytochrome P450 and extragonadal estrogen play a role in ischemic neuroprotection. *J. Neurosci.* 23:8701-8705, 2003

[42] MacMahon B: Risk factors for endometrial cancer. *Gynecol. Oncol.* 2:122-129, 1974

[43] Massarweh S, Schiff R: Resistance to endocrine therapy in breast cancer: exploiting estrogen receptor/growth factor crosstalk. *Endocrin-Related Cancer Suppl.* 13, 1:S15-24, 2006

[44] Massarweh S, Osborne CK, CreightonCJ, Qin L, Tsimelson A, Huang S, Weiss H, Rimawl M, Schiff R: Tamoxifen resistance in breast tumors is driven by growth factor receptor signaling with repression of classic estrogen receptor genomic function. *Cancer Res.* 68:826-833, 2008

[45] Miller WR, O'Neill J: The importance of local synthesis of estrogen within the breast. *Steroids* 50:537-548, 1987

[46] Muti P, Quattrin T, Grant BJB et al: Fasting glucose is a risk factor for breast cancer. *Cancer Epidemiol. Biomark and Prev.* 11:1361-1368, 2002

[47] Nand SL, Webster MA, Baber R. The Oestrogen/Provera Study Group. Bleeding pattern and the endometrial changes during continuous combined hormone replacement therapy. *Obstet Gynecol.* 91:678-684, 1998

[48] Negri E, Tzonou A, Beral V, Trichopoulos D, Parazzini F, Franceschi S, Booth M, LaVecchia C: Hormonal therapy for menopause and ovarian cancer in a collaborative re-analysis of European studies. *Int. J. Cancer* 80:848-851, 1999

[49] Nestler JE, Strauss JF: Insulin as an effector of human ovarian and adrenal steroid metabolism. *Endocrin. Metab. Clin. North Amer.* 20:807-823, 1991

[50] Olsson H, Jernström H, Alm P, Kreipe H, Ingvar C, Jönsson PE, Rydén S: Proliferation of the breast epithelium in relation to menstrual cycle phase, hormonal use, and reproductive factors. *Breast Cancer Res. Treat* 40:187-196, 1996

[51] Olsson H, Bladström AM, Ingvar C: Are smoking-associated cancers prevented or postponed in women using hormone replacement therapy? *Obstet Gynecol.* 102:565-570, 2003

[52] Parazzini F, La Vecchia C, Negri E, Franceschi S, Bolis G: Case-control study of estrogen replacement therapy and risk of cervical cancer. *British Med. J.* 315:85-88, 1997

[53] Parvez S, Tabassum H, Banerjee BD, Raisuddin S: Taurine prevents tamoxifen-induced mitochondrial oxidative damage in mice. *Basic and Clinical Pharmacol and Toxicol* 102:382-387, 2008

[54] Pierpoint T, McKeigue PM, Isaacs AJ, Wild SH, Jacobs HS: Mortality of women with polycystic ovary syndrome at long-term follow-up. *J. Clin. Epidemiol.* 51:581-586, 1998

[55] Pillay OC, Te Fong LF, Crow JC, Benjamin E, Mould T, Atiomo W, Menon PA, Leonard AJ, Hardiman P: The association between polycystic ovaries and endometrial cancer. *Human Reprod.* 21:924-929, 2006

[56] Polson DW, Wadsworth J, Adams J et al: Polycystic ovaries: a common finding in normal women. *Lancet* 1:870-872, 1988

[57] Risch HA: Hormone replacement therapy and the risk of ovarian cancer. *Gynecol. Oncol.* 86:115-117, 2002

[58] Rodriguez C, Patel AV, Calle EE, Jakob EJ: Estrogen replacement therapy and ovarian cancer mortality in a large prospective study of US women. *J. Am. Med. Assoc.* 285:1460-1465, 2001

[59] Rodriguez C, Feigelson HS, Deka A, Patel AV, Jacobs EJ, Thun MJ, Calle EE: Postmenopausal hormone therapy and lung cancer risk in the Cancer Prevention Study II Nutrition Cohort. *Cancer Epidemiol. Biomark and Prev.* 17:655-660, 2008

[60] Santen RJ, Martel J, Hoagland M, Naftolin F, Roa L, Harada N, Hafer L, Zaino R, Santner SJ: Stromal spindle cells contain aromatase in human breast-tumors. *J. Clin. Endocrin. Metab.* 79:627-632, 1994

[61] Sartor BM, Dickey RP: Polycystic ovarian syndrome and the metabolic syndrome. *Am. J. Med.* 330:336-342, 2005

[62] Schapiro S: False alarm: postmenopausal hormone therapy and ovarian cancer. *Climacteric* 10:466-470, 2007

[63] Shackney SE, McCormack GW, Jr Cuchural GJ: Growth rate patterns of solid tumors and their relation to responsiveness to therapy: an analytical review. *Ann. Intern. Med.* 89:107-121, 1978

[64] Sitruk-Warre R: Progestogens in hormonal replacement therapy: New molecules, risks and benefits. *Menopause* 9:6-15, 2002

[65] Smith EP, Boyd J, Frank GR, Takahashi H, Cohen RM, Specker B et al: Estrogen resistance caused by a mutation in the estrogen receptor gene in a man. *New Engl. J. Med.* 331:1056-1061, 1994

[66] Soliman PT, Oh JC, Schmeler KM, Sun CC, Slomovitz BM, Gershenson DM, Burke TW, Lu KH: Risk factors for young premenopausal women with endometrial cancer. *Obstet Gynecol.* 105:575-580, 2005

[67] Spratt JS, Spratt JA: What is breast cancer doing before we can detect it? *J. Surg. Oncol.* 30:156-160, 1985

[68] Spratt JS, Meyer JS, Spratt JA: Rates of growth of human solid neoplasms: part I. J. *Surg. Oncol.* 60:137-146, 1995

[69] Spritzer PM, Morsch DM, Wiltgen D: Polycystic ovary syndrome associated neoplasms. Arq. Bras Endocrinol. Metabol. 49:805-810, 2006

[70] Suba Zs: Gender-related hormonal risk factors for oral cancer. Pathol Oncol. Res. 13:195-202, 2007

[71] Suba Zs: Systemic risk factors for oral cancer: Estrogen deficiency and insulin resistance. Chapter 8. pp: 157-172 In: Progress in Oral Cancer Research. Ed: Frederik L. Nielsen, Nova Science Publishers, 2008

[72] Varras M, Polyzos D, Akviris C: Effects of tamoxifen on the human female genital tract: Review of the literature. *Eur. J. Gynaecol. Oncol.* 24:258-268, 2003

[73] Van Landeghem AAJ, Poortman J, Nabuurs M, Thijssen JH: Endogenous concentration and subcellular distribution of estrogens in normal and malignant breast tissue. *Cancer Res.* 45:2900-2906, 1985

[74] Weiderpass E, Gridley G, Persson I et al: Risk of endometrial and breast cancer in patients with diabetes mellitus. *Int. J. Cancer* 71:360-363, 1997

[75] Whittemore AS, Harris R, Itnyre J: Characteristics relating to ovarian cancer risk: collaborative analysis of 12 US case-control studies. IL Invasive epithelial ovarian cancers in white women. Collaborative Ovarian Cancer Group. *Am. J. Epidemiol.* 136: 1184-1203, 1992

[76] WHO Classification on Pathology and Genetics In Tavassoli FA, Devile P(eds): Tumours of the Breast and Female Genital Organs. WHO Publications, Geneva, Switzerland. 2003

[77] Wisemann RA: Brest cancer hypothesis: a single cause for the majority of cases. *J. Epidemiol. Community Haelth* 54:851-858, 2000

Chapter 7

Insulin Resistance, Estrogen Deficiency and Cancer Risk

The Diabolic Triad

Insulin resistance and estrogen deficiency are well-known concordant disorders with mutual interrelationship. Moderate or severe estrogen deficiency proved to be a high risk factor for insulin resistance both in premenopausal and postmenopausal women as well as in rare male cases [9,31,59]. On the other hand insulin resistance and hyperinsulinemia provoke a severe imbalance in sexual steroid synthesis resulting in excessive androgen and low estrogen levels and interferes with estrogen effect even at receptor level [70].

Our knowledge concerning consequences of insulin resistance is relatively young; its multifaceted complications were revealed at the end of the 20th century and at the same time it was regarded as a high risk for hypertension and arteriosclerotic lesions (see Chapter 2). Recognition of correlations between insulin resistance and malignancies suffered several years' delay, but recently the role of insulin resistance in initiation and progression of cancer has been undoubtedly justified. On the contrary, estrogen deficiency had been a traditional etiologic factor for postmenopausal cardiovascular diseases for a long time. Now, after a long delay it is time for estrogen deficiency to join cancer risk factors (Figure 7.1).

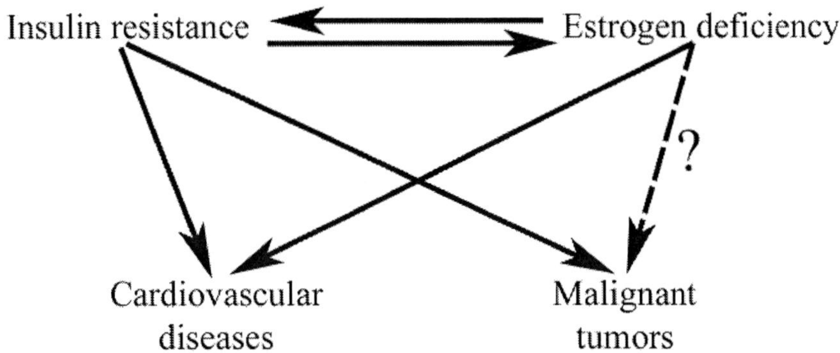

Figure 7.1. Correlations between insulin resistance, estrogen deficiency and their complications.

Clinical Associations between Estrogen Deficiency and Insulin Resistance

A moderate or severe decrease of female steroid hormone levels enhances the prevalence of insulin resistant states both in premenopausal and postmenopausal cases. Clinical investigations suggest that *in premenopausal women* long or highly irregular menstrual cycles are predictors for risk of type-2 diabetes [85]. Consequently, estrogen deficiency affects not only the generative functions but also the general health of women.

The polycystic ovarium syndrome (PCOS) in young, premenopausal women is an important pathologic example of the correlations between estrogen deficiency and insulin resistance [9]. The cardinal symptoms are anovulation, infertility, hirsutism and obesity. In the background insulin resistance, hyperinsulinism and hyperandrogenism are the main findings [70]. The luteinizing hormone may also be increased and in typical cases decreased levels of sex hormone binding and IGF-I binding proteins may be found.

In PCOS cases insulin resistance and hyperinsulinemia overregulate ovarian androgen synthesis at the expense of reduction of estrogen production [71]. In young PCOS cases the deceiving presentation of normal serum glucose level and regular cycles may be insidiously associated with severe hyperinsulinemia and laboratory findings of hyperandrogenism [17].

The use of insulin sensitizing drugs in PCOS cases has been shown to lower serum insulin level, which improves many of the troublesome manifestations of the syndrome. Metformin is the most commonly used insulin level lowering drug in PCOS cases and it can improve menstrual abnormalities, ovulatory dysfunction, infertility and hirsutism [71]. However, in the rare cases of estrogen deficient males the severe type-2 diabetes may be treated by estrogen administration [31].

Women with PCOS have been shown to have consistently higher rates of metabolic syndrome [35,80,81]. Among women with PCOS diagnosis the prevalence of metabolic syndrome was evaluated to be 43%. This represents a twofold higher prevalence than that reported for age-matched women in the general population [1].

In PCOS cases increased prevalence and predictors of risk for impaired glucose tolerance and type-2 diabetes were assessed in prospective controlled studies [53]. Impaired glucose tolerance was observed in 20 to 40% of women with PCOS, which was a significantly higher prevalence than among age and weight-matched premenopausal women. Type-2 diabetes proved to be three to seven times more likely to develop in women with PCOS as compared with control patients [53,28]. In young women PCOS may predict an increased risk of both metabolic syndrome and type-2 diabetes [28,29,35,53]. Similarly, among premenopausal women with type-2 diabetes, an increased prevalence of PCOS could be observed [73].

Adolescent girls with PCOS have profound metabolic derangement detected early in the course of the syndrome including insulin resistance and compensatory hyperinsulinemia. These observations predict an increased risk for type-2 diabetes of PCOS cases even in adolescence [54].

PCOS is not an infertility disease alone but is a systemic disorder with long-term consequences. PCOS associated insulin resistance means general health risks for the affected women. Increased prevalence of diabetes mellitus, hypertension and cardiac complications were observed in a follow up study of a Dutch population of women with PCOS [29]. Close associations between PCOS and premature coronary and aortic atherosclerosis were revealed in middle-aged women [90,91]. A retrospective Swedish study found 7.4-fold risk of myocardial infarction among women suffering of PCOS [24]. Correlation between polycystic ovaries and extent of coronary artery disease was justified in women having cardiac catheterization [7]. However, another study on the general health of PCOS cases could not justify a significantly increased rate of cardiovascular mortality among women with PCOS as compared with that of the general female population [74].

Elevated androgen levels in women are also associated with an increased risk of type-2 diabetes [96]. Excessive androgen level may be due to the decreased conversion of testosterone to estrogen by aromatase cytochrome P450 resulting in decreased estrogen level [4]. When the ratio of androgen/estrogen level is increased in women, development of male physical characteristics of muscle mass and android type visceral adipose tissue accumulations are the most important symptoms. Such women have an increased risk of developing hypertension, type-2 diabetes and cardiovascular disease [8]. The mechanism may be muscular insulin resistance in women with relative androgen excess.

In the *climacteric and postmenopausal period*, increased body weight and central body fat distribution are often observed in women and the prevalences of type-2 diabetes and impaired glucose tolerance increase dramatically with age [52]. Theories emerged that estrogen deficiency and increased androgen activity are responsible for the worsening of glucose homeostasis in genetically susceptible postmenopausal women [40,97]. Among postmenopausal women serum glucose and insulin levels have been found to be higher than among premenopausal patients, and increased prevalence of metabolic syndrome and type-2 diabetes have also been observed after menopause [32,81,98].

Earlier literary data on the relationship between menopause and type-2 diabetes are more or less controversial. Several authors showed that there is no significant correlation between changes in fasting plasma glucose level and natural or surgical menopause [10,44,59]. Recently, postmenopausal estrogen deficiency appears to be associated with an increased risk for development of the metabolic syndrome [81]. Moreover, menopause appeared to be an important risk factor for diabetes in Japanese-American women as it was associated with accumulation of visceral fat and development of insulin resistance [33].

A possible explanation for these conflicting observations is that researchers did not consider age at menopause and years following the onset of menopause in the examined cases [98]. Glucose and insulin levels as well as insulin sensitivity might not change immediately following menopause. However, a progressive increase was seen in insulin resistance and in serum insulin levels that relate to time since menopause rather than to chronological age of the patients [36,77]. This continuous progression of insulin resistance in postmenopausal women suggests a close correlation with the decreasing ovarian estrogen production.

Comparison of pre- and postmenopausal women exhibited a 2.3-fold increase in impaired glucose tolerance and a 5.7-fold increase in type-2 diabetes in the latter group. Every year after menopause conferred a negative influence on insulin sensitivity and increased the risk of impaired glucose tolerance [98]. Glucose intolerance in postmenopausal women has been consistently reported as risk factor for cardiovascular diseases [38]. It is very important for clinical practitioners to take glucose intolerance into consideration in women with increasing number of years after menopause.

Molecular Mechanism of Estrogen Effect on Glucose Metabolism

Estrogen has beneficial effects on the energy metabolism and glucose homeostasis by means of several possible pathways [5]. It regulates the insulin production capacity of the pancreatic islet cells [22]. In the liver, estrogen regulates insulin sensitivity by the activation of glycogen synthase and glycolytic enzymes [13]. Moreover, estrogen advantageously regulates the activity of glucose transporters in the peripheral target tissues [14].

Elevated plasma glucose level during the post-prandial phase is controlled by increased insulin secretion of the pancreatic β-cells. In animal experiments ovarectomy is associated with increased risk of diabetes, whereas estrogen administration improves the insulin response to glucose load [37]. Estrogen enhanced glucose-induced insulin secretion within 3-5 minutes of perfusion into whole rat pancreas and in mouse islets [22,37]. The mechanism is not fully clarified, but estrogen appears to act synergistically with glucose resulting in a calcium-mediated stimulation of insulin secretion. This may explain the apparent suppression of glucose induced insulin secretion in estrogen deficiency.

In aromatase knockout (ArKO) mice the enzyme for estrogen biosynthesis is inactivated, and these estrogen deficient animals have reduced glucose oxidation, increased adiposity and high insulin levels, which are the features of insulin resistance. Glucose intolerance of ArKO mice can be reversed by estrogen treatment both in females and males [47]!

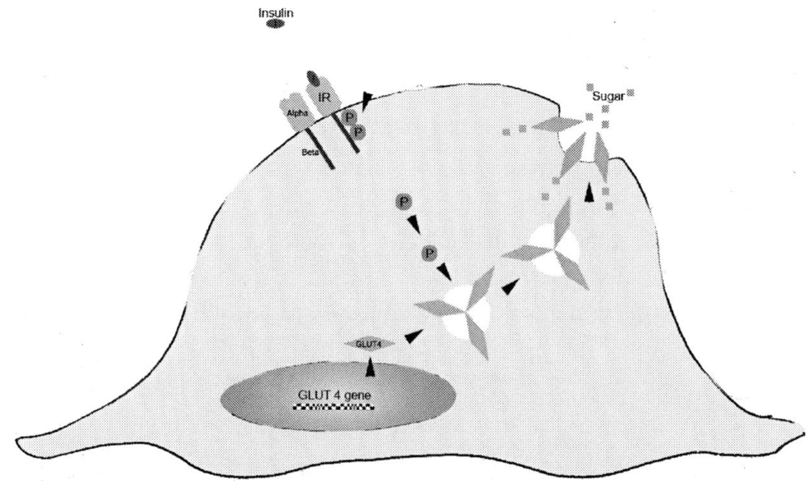

Correlation between Insulin Receptor and Glucose transporters

I - Insulin; IR - Insulin Receptor (Alpha-Beta dimer); GLUT4 - Glucose transporter

Source: Barros RPA, Machado UF and Gustafsson JA: Trends in Molecular Medicine 9:425-431, 2006.

Figure 7.2. Model summarizing the interaction of insulin and glucose uptake in insulin-sensitive tissues. Insulin receptors are located on the cell membrane and their activation by the hormone causes the phosphorylation of the transmembrane subunit b. Once activated, several cytoplasmatic proteins are phosphorylated, including IRS-1 and PI3-K, which are essential for insulin signaling. The end result of this phosphorylation cascade is the translocation of vesicles that contain GLUT4 to the cell membrane, where the protein anchors and enables the uptake of glucose by facilitated diffusion. Any alteration in insulin signaling (1), GLUT4 expression (2), translocation or anchorage (3) causes insulin resistance. Abbreviations: GLUT4, glucose transporter 4; IRS-1, insulin receptor substrate 1; P, phosphate; PI3-K, phosphatidylinositol 3-kinase.

In estrogen deficient states, such as menopause, increased prevalence of type-2 diabetes and obesity may be only partially reversed by restricted diet because it cannot improve pancreatic β-cell mass and function. However, in postmenopausal women regular physical activity or even estrogen replacement alone has more beneficial metabolic effect suggesting their direct impact on improving insulin secretion capacity and proliferation of β-cells [22]. Consequently, estrogen treatment in postmenopausal women may prevent the prevalence of type-2 diabetes and delay its progression.

In the liver, glucose homeostasis is maintained by the equilibrium of glycogen synthesis and glycogenolysis. Insulin regulates the glucose uptake and glucose output of the liver in case of normal insulin sensitivity [5]. Abnormalities of the enzyme activities in the liver can lead to insulin resistance. In ER-α receptor knockout (ERKO) animals [56] hepatic insulin resistance is associated with decreased glucose uptake in skeletal muscles [13]. These findings reveal evidence that estrogen receptor-alpha plays an important role in the regulation of glucose homeostasis and of insulin sensitivity of the liver in mice.

Peripheral glucose uptake requires an active transport through the double lipid layer of the cell membrane (Figure 7.2). Insulin binding to the insulin receptors on the cell surface is the first step to transport glucose molecules to the cytoplasm. Insulin receptors have two α-subunits, which are located on the outer surface of the cell and contain the binding sites for insulin, whereas the two transmembrane β-subunits are responsible for signal transduction.

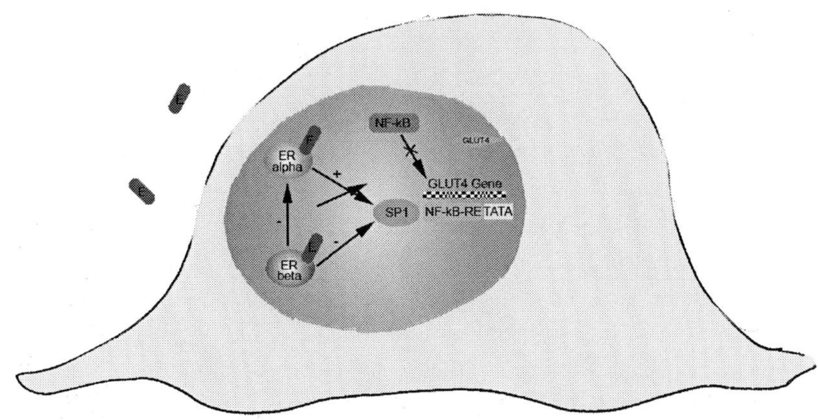

Correlations between Estrogen Receptors and Glucose transporters

ER - Estrogen Receptor (Alpha or Beta); NFkB - Nuclear Factor kB

GLUT4 - Glucose transporter; NFkB-RE - NFkB Responsive Element; TATA - TATA Box

Source: Barros RPA, Machado UF and Gustafsson JA: Trends in Molecular Medicine 9:425-431, 2006.

Figure 7.3. Model representing mechanisms by which ERa and ERb might modulate expression of the gene that encodes GLUT4. E2 exerts its action through ERa and ERb, which interact with the promoter region of the gene through transcriptional factors SP1 and NF-kB. The activation of ERa increases protein expression through SP1, a stimulator of GLUT4 expression. ERa also inhibits the binding of NF-kB to its response element. NF-kB is a potent repressor of GLUT4 expression and this inhibition might lead to increased GLUT4 expression. In contrast, activation of ERb opposes ERa action and inhibits SP1-induced gene expression, reducing GLUT4 content. Abbreviations: ERa, estrogen receptor a; ERb, estrogen receptor b; GLUT4, glucose transporter 4; NF-kB, nuclear factor-kB; NF-kB -RE, nuclear factor kB response element; SP1, specificity protein 1; TATA box, initiation site of transcription.

When insulin interacts with the external α-subunits, autophosphorylation of the β-subunits occurs at multiple tyrosines, which results in activation of insulin signal transduction [50]. This phosphorylation cascade provokes translocation of glucose transporter (GLUT4) containing cytoplasmic vesicles to the cell membrane [99]. GLUT4 anchored to the cell membrane enables the facilitated diffusion of glucose from the extracellular space into the cell [39]. Any alteration in these mechanisms, such as insulin signal transduction, GLUT4 expression and/or translocation may result in insulin resistance [5].

Estrogen receptors (ERs) are newly recognized important players in glucose metabolism [5]. They advantageously modulate insulin stimulated glucose uptake through regulation of the tyrosine phosphorylation of insulin receptor protein [64].

ERs have crucial roles in peripheral glucose uptake by regulation of glucose transporters (Figure 7.3). They participate both in GLUT4 expression and translocation. In ovarectomized rats, estradiol substitution increased the amount of GLUT1 protein in the blood-brain barrier [83]. In immature rat uterus estradiol treatment caused a fourfold increase in GLUT1 protein content and also increased glucose uptake [95]. In another study expression of GLUT1, GLUT3 and GLUT4 decreased in the frontal cortex of castrated female monkeys, however, estradiol treatment reversed the glucose transporter expression in the cortical tissue [19].

In human adipocytes GLUT4 abundance is highly correlated with insulin responsiveness. In PCOS cases, in which ovarian overproduction of testosterone is characteristic, insulin stimulated glucose uptake was reduced due to decreased amounts of GLUT4 on adipocyte membrane [79].

However, studies on ovarectomized rats revealed that high doses of estradiol alone or in combination with progesterone decreased GLUT4 expression in the adipose tissue [89]. Another study showed that physiological doses of estradiol and progesterone reduced GLUT4 expression in the smooth muscle and white adipose tissue of ovarectomized rats [14]. However, this reduction might also be attributed to reduced physical activity of these animals and not only to the administered hormones [5].

ER-α and ER-β seem to have opposite actions on glucose homeostasis and modulation of GLUT4 activities. Mice that lack ER-α are insulin resistant; exhibit impaired glucose tolerance and obesity, affecting both males and females. This highlights the importance of ER-α action for maintenance of normal glucose homeostasis in both sexes [42]. In contrast, the role of ER-β in this homeostasis has not been perfectly clarified. In mice that lack ER-α, estradiol retrieval by ovarectomy improved the glucose metabolism [66], suggesting that ER-β activation might have a diabetogenic effect and opposes the action of ER-α [5]. In mice, GLUT4 regulation in the gastrocnemius muscle by both estrogen receptor isoforms is a further important proof for correlations between ERs and regulation of insulin sensitivity [5].

A plausible hypothesis is that in cells with coexpression of both ER isoforms there is a continuously adjusted balance between ER-α and ER-β to maintain the ideal GLUT4 expression and glucose homeostasis.

Estradiol regulates the action of insulin at receptor level in a concentration-specific manner [67]. Higher concentrations of estradiol can inhibit insulin signaling by modulation of insulin receptor substrate-1 (IRS-l) phosphorylation in 3T3-Ll adipocytes. As insulin has not only metabolic but also mitogenic effects, inhibition of the excessive insulin receptor signal by estrogen may be a safety impact both against pathological glucose uptake and cell proliferation.

Summarizing the effects of estrogen and ER signals, they are important regulators of glucose uptake and insulin sensitivity and have mainly antidiabetogenic impacts. In vitro studies, animal experiments and clinical examinations justify that estrogen deficiency or disturbances in the ER signal result in insulin resistance, even type-2 diabetes.

Effects of Estrogen on Lipid Metabolism

Hypercholesterolemia, high level of low-density lipoprotein (LDL) and low level of high-density lipoprotein (HDL) cholesterol concentrations of the serum mean high risk factors for atherosclerosis and its complications (see Chapter 4). Postmenopausal women have higher total cholesterol, LDL cholesterol and triglyceride levels and lower HDL cholesterol levels compared with premenopausal women. These changes may be regarded as a shift toward a more atherogenic lipid profile in postmenopausal cases [46].

Postmenopausal estrogen therapy may reduce the risk of cardiovascular disease and this beneficial effect may be mediated in part by favorable changes in plasma lipid levels. Oral estradiol treatment reduced the LDL cholesterol concentrations by its accelerated catabolism while minimalizing the potentially adverse effects on triglyceride levels [94].

In animal experiments, estradiol administration lowered the level of lipid peroxidation and improved the dysfunction parameters of the liver in aged rats [41]. The LDL receptor (LDLR) gene is activated by estradiol in the liver, which suggests an important role of estrogen in hepatic lipid metabolism [55]. The non-genomic tyrosine kinase signaling system was also shown to have important impact on estrogen-induced LDL receptor gene expression in HepG2 cells [27]. Furthermore, an androgen receptor-mediated antagonism of estrogen-dependent LDLR transcription was observed in cultured hepatocytes [23]. This observation may at least partially reveal the antagonistic associations of sexual steroids with lipid metabolism and vascular diseases.

Effects of Insulin on Steroid Hormone Production and on their Signals at Receptor Level

Among premenopausal, young women with type-2 diabetes 25-28% exhibited the clinical evidence of PCOS and the associated imbalance of the sexual hormone levels [73]. Moreover, in young women with type-2 diabetes the prevalence of polycystic ovaries proved to be as high as 80% after thorough investigations [21].

Insulin is a potent effector of human sexual steroid hormone production in the endocrine organs and modulates estrogen signals at receptor level. Insulin resistance may contribute to hyperandrogenism and anovulatory dysfunction through several pathways [80]. Furthermore, insulin and insulin-like growth factor receptors transfer potent mitogenic stimuli and share important functions with ERs in the control of cellular proliferation. Interplays among insulin, IGF and estrogen receptor signals are discussed in Chapter 5.

Hyperinsulinemia in the first, compensated phase of insulin resistance stimulates ovarian androgen production at the expense of reduction of estrogen synthesis [70]. Elevated insulin level stimulates testosterone biosynthesis of human ovarian thecal cells from women with PCOS. Thus hyperinsulinemia results in a serious imbalance of sexual steroid hormone levels, by causing an excess of androgens and estrogen deficiency. After therapeutic reduction of insulin secretion in PCOS cases a decrease in ovarian cytochrome P450c17 alpha activity and serum free testosterone level could be observed [69]. Treatment by insulin sensitizing Metformin was shown to inhibit directly the androgen overproduction in human ovarian thecal cells [2].

Insulin and insulin-like growth factor-I receptors may synergize with luteinizing hormone (LH) to promote androgen production by ovarian theca cells [15,16]. Further evidences supported that increased androgen production by ovarian theca cells in PCOS cases may be caused by an additional intrinsic alteration in their steroidogenic activity [68]. Insulin may also affect the pituitary to favor the secretion of LH and increases adrenal androgen production by means of an increased adrenal sensitivity to adrenocorticotropin [61]. Insulin, somatotropin and luteinizing hormone axes may also have gonadotropin augmenting effects both in lean and obese PCOS cases, resulting in endocrine and metabolic dysfunctions [63]. Hyperfunction of the hypothalamic-pituitary axis in women with PCOS was also justified as causal factor of altered neuroendocrine regulation of gonadotropin secretion [92,93].

Increased Cancer Risk of Insulin Resistance among Women as Compared with Men

Gender-related differences in all cause and cardiovascular mortality were observed related to hyperglycemia and newly diagnosed diabetes (45). Several literary data suggest that insulin resistance is a higher cancer risk for women than for men, especially after menopause (see Chapter 3). As insulin resistance is a proven risk for cancer initiation and progression, the associated estrogen deficiency may cause even higher cancer risk. Pre- or postmenopausal decrease of estrogen level, relative excess of androgens and hyperinsulinemia with the concomitantly elevated IGF-I level exert a cross fire at cellular level and may induce serious gene alterations, even malignant transformation.

In Sweden type-2 diabetes and insulin resistance were established as cancer risks preferentially in women. The total cancer risk in women significantly increased with rising plasma levels of fasting and postload glucose, however in men this correlation was not observed [87].

In a study in India, associations between diabetes mellitus and premalignant oral lesions, such as leukoplakia and erythroplakia were observed only in female cases, although the underlying mechanisms were not discussed [26]. In a representative sample of the US population diabetes was found as an independent predictor for oral leukoplakia. However, postmenopausal female cases with a history of estrogen use were less likely to have oral leukoplakia with an OR of 0.34 [25]. These data justify the defending effect of HRT use against oral premalignancies.

Among Hungarian oral cancer cases, elevated fasting glucose proved to be a significantly high cancer risk among near exclusively postmenopausal women but not in men. These results suggest that insulin resistance and estrogen deficiency are combined cancer risk factors in women [88].

Correlations between glycemic index and glycemic load as well as risk for upper aerodigestive tract neoplasms were also studied [3]. The risk was apparently stronger in women with high body mass index and insulin resistance as compared with men. Though exact data on the menopausal state of female cases were not published, cancers at these sites affect typically older women. Consequently, obese, insulin resistant postmenopausal women with lower estrogen levels exhibited increased inclination to oral and pharyngeal cancers associated with high glycemic load.

Cancer of the gingival tissue has a unique position among cancers. Though gingiva shows well-known high estrogen sensitivity, its cancer occurs both in male and female patients. Nevertheless, gingival cancer exhibits a conspicuously higher prevalence among women as compared with men. In our Hungarian case control studies strikingly increased prevalence of gingival cancer among postmenopausal women was observed as compared with men [88]. High prevalence of gingival cancer among postmenopausal women with elevated fasting glucose also justified the carcinogenic capacity of combined estrogen deficiency and insulin resistance on highly hormone sensitive tissues in female cases.

The squamous epithelial cell lining of the oral cavity and squamous oral cancer cells have more or less estrogen and progesterone receptors, which justifies that these tumors may be moderately hormone dependent [62]. Assessment of sexual hormone receptor status of oral, laryngeal and hypopharyngeal cancers revealed a predominance of ER alpha expression, however, sexual hormone receptor expressions did not affect the survival of patients [57]. Further similar studies would be necessary to compare the sexual hormone receptor expression of oral cancers between male and female patients, especially in gingival cancer cases.

Increased Cancer Risk of Insulin Resistance among Postmenopausal as Compared with Premenopausal Cases

There are many literary data to support that both pre- and postmenopausal estrogen deficiency are associated with insulin resistance [28,29,36,81,99]. Considering the cancer risk factors, different grades of estrogen deficiency and the associated insulin resistance have pivotal role in the development of malignancies in pre- and postmenopausal women.

However, cancer epidemiology shows quite different features depending on the hormonal status of women. In premenopausal women marked prevalence of cancers in the highly hormone sensitive organs may be observed, whereas in postmenopausal cases the cancer incidence of both highly and moderately estrogen sensitive organs shows an increasing trend.

The tumor incidence rate of the moderately estrogen sensitive organs is low in premenopausal cases, and increases slowly after menopause in middle-aged women and steeply in elderly women over 60 years of age (see in Chapter 6). As oral cancer is a typical example of the moderately estrogen sensitive tumors, its initiation usually requires a profound estrogen deficiency, especially in the absence of other, exogenous noxae.

Our Hungarian epidemiological study on oral cancer cases resulted in a disclosure of two systemic risk factors for oral cancer, namely, estrogen deficiency and elevated fasting glucose in postmenopausal women [88]. Smoking and excessive alcohol consumption proved to be strong but not exclusive risk factors for oral cancer among these women. These two risk factors have not only harmful local effects, but they may also induce complex mechanisms affecting disadvantageously the metabolic and hormonal system. Smoking and excessive alcohol consumption have close interrelations with insulin resistance, enhanced oxidative stress and increased ratio of male to female sexual steroid levels. These systemic changes may exert their carcinogenic capacity on the oral mucosa in a second phase via the circulatory system.

Among young, premenopausal women even slight or moderate estrogen deficiency may induce gene regulation disorders preferentially in the highly estrogen sensitive organs. In premenopausal women PCOS with anovulation and insulin resistance means a common risk for cancers of the breast, endometrium and ovary [34]. Mortality data of women with PCOS were examined in a long-term follow up study in the UK and breast cancer was the most common cause of deaths [74].

A strong association between PCOS and endometrial cancer was also observed and this was confined preferentially to premenopausal women [75]. In a further study nulliparity, irregular or long menstrual cycles, diabetes and hypertension were strongly associated with endometrial cancer and in addition a high incidence of synchronous primary ovarian cancers could be observed in premenopausal cases [84]. Primary ovarian cancers are also frequently associated with PCOS in young women [74,86].

Insulin resistance seemed to be decisive risk factor for endometrial cancer, and this correlation proved to be independent of endogenous hormone levels of the patients [76]. In an Italian case-control study, correlations of diet with ovarian cancer were assessed [11]. A diet giving defence against insulin resistance, including fish, raw and cooked vegetables as well as pulses showed an inverse association with cancer risk of the ovary. Unfortunately, hormonal disorders and menopausal state of the women included in the study were not registered.

Breast cancer may be regarded as a typical example of tumors of highly hormone sensitive organs. Recently, in a prospective study, correlations of fasting serum glucose level and breast cancer risk were examined separately in pre- and postmenopausal women [65]. This study allowed for distinction between patients with different estrogen levels. Elevated fasting glucose was a significant tumor predictor in both groups of breast cancer cases. Moreover, elevated serum levels of bioavailable free and protein bound IGF-I also showed correlation with breast cancer risk both in pre- and postmenopausal cases, especially among obese older women! Postmenopausal obesity was associated with a higher risk of breast cancer, particularly among women not using hormone replacement, whereas obese premenopausal women had a lower breast cancer risk [65].

However, the authors did not discuss their striking but absolutely correct finding that a postmenopausal HRT proved to be beneficial against breast cancer risk. These results reflect in an exact manner that insulin resistance alone in hormonally active premenopausal women is not so high breast cancer risk as compared with combined insulin resistance and estrogen deficiency in postmenopausal cases without HRT use.

In a recent study, breast cancer incidence in women diagnosed at or after age of 65 years showed strong positive association with highly elevated fasting blood glucose (> or =7.0 mmol/l) [78]. In these elderly women, at least 15 years after the average age of menopause, combination of severe estrogen deficiency and insulin resistance were strong, combined risk factors for breast cancer.

Obesity and insulin resistance in postmenopausal women exhibit increased prevalence [81,98] and they are obviously associated with increased ratio of male to female sexual steroids and estrogen deficiency. Clinical studies support that type-2 diabetes also shows close correlations with an excessive androgen level in women [96]. Taken together, increased cancer risk due to insulin resistance and hyperinsulinemia among endangered postmenopausal women would require no further justification, however these disorders are associated with elevated androgen and decreased estrogen levels [40].

Literary data on the hormonal and metabolic background of postmenopausal breast cancer cases present many controversial associations. Obesity, insulin resistance and type-2 diabetes proved to be unquestionable risk factors for breast cancer among postmenopausal women [12,43,60], though these findings are associated typically with estrogen deficiency. Moreover, an abnormal androgen production was exhibited in women with breast cancers [82]. These correlations contradict to the coexistence of insulin resistance and excessive estrogen level, which are regarded as common risk factors for breast cancer.

Though literary data on breast cancer risk struggle with the metabolic and hormonal contradictions the principle of estrogen carcinogenicity seems to be irrefutable. Many authors stand up for the carcinogenic capacity of estrogen in postmenopausal breast cancer cases [6,49,51,72]. Moreover, the main therapeutic measures include antiestrogen treatment against excessive, "harmful" estrogen effect in postmenopausal women. However, if the researcher insists on the premise that increased estrogen level is associated with breast cancer risk, the antagonism between insulin resistance and estrogen excess remains to be solved.

Several authors tried to reconcile the contradictions between high serum androgen levels and breast cancer risk with preservation of the idea of estrogen carcinogenicity [30,51,58].

In clinical studies, concomitantly elevated serum estradiol and testosterone concentrations were found to be associated with breast cancer risk [18,51], which seem to be controversial. Carcinogenic capacity of estrogen in postmenopausal women was also supported by the surprising assumption that adrenal androgens may stimulate the proliferation of breast cancer cells as direct activators of estrogen receptor-α [58]. Moreover, increased body mass index and fat deposition in insulin resistant, postmenopausal cases raised the idea of excessive conversion of testosterone to estrogen by aromatase activity of adipocytes [48]. All these ideas favoured to the evidence of estrogen induced breast cancer risk in postmenopausal women.

Recently, postmenopausal estrogen production of cells in different organs with high estrogen demand, such as endothelium, glia, bone, breast and endometrium evoked many controversies and debates. This extraovarian estrogen accumulation may serve as a defence for organs, which exhibit enhanced vulnerability in estrogen deficient milieu rather than as a newly formed possibility to access chronic diseases, even cancers (see Chapter 5).

Interestingly, the wide spread use of antiestrogen therapy against ER-positive breast cancers has severe side effects affecting the organs with high estrogen demand. Increased prevalence of malignancies of the endometrium and ischemic injury of the central nervous system as complications of tamoxifen treatment have been published (see Chapter 6).

A further important question is the definition of "elevated serum estrogen concentration" in postmenopausal women. Dangerously elevated estrogen level in postmenopausal patients seems to be an absurdity even in case of HRT use. Epidemiological studies on breast cancer cases include pooled populations of postmenopausal cases. However, during the postmenopausal period the estrogen level decreases continuously, steeply or mildly. The normal range of estrogen levels cannot be estimated without taking into consideration the years after menopause and age of the patient. Supposedly, the longer the postmenopausal period of a patient the lower her serum estrogen level. A more informative investigation would be to compare the estrogen levels of women with and without breast cancer 1-2 years and 10-15 years after menopause.

Importance of Combined Insulin Resistance and Estrogen Deficiency as Cancer Risk

Summarising the dangers of combined insulin resistance and estrogen deficiency as cancer risk, conspicuous differences can be found between male and female patients.

Estrogen predominance against androgens in healthy women is a favour in their reproductive period, which means a strong defence against both cardiovascular lesions and malignant tumors. However, at the same time, high estrogen demand of all female tissues, especially breast and gynaecological organs, means an increased cancer risk in estrogen deficient states both in pathological premenopausal and physiological postmenopausal cases. This disadvantage of estrogen deficient women is evident when considering a population with insulin resistance or type-2 diabetes, they have a higher risk for precancerous lesions and cancers as compared with men.

Complete estrogen lack in male cases is extraordinarily rare and is associated with severe form of type-2 diabetes [31]. Such men may be well treated by estrogen substitution. The rarity of these cases makes impossible to assess the risk for cardiovascular diseases or malignancies of complete estrogen deficiency in men.

However, an increased ratio of the male to female sexual hormone levels can be induced by anabolic steroid treatment of young sportsmen and its association with insulin resistance could be justified [20]. Recently, occurrence of unexplained, sudden cardiac death among leading young sportsmen could be attributed mainly to artificially induced anabolic androgen excess and relative estrogen deficiency. As clinical cancer development from its initiation takes many years, assessment of cancer incidence among inactive sportsmen would be a possibility for disclosure of the late complications of androgen excess and estrogen deficiency in men.

Cancer incidence in elderly cases is not unusual, however, unexpected cancer exhibition in young or middle-aged patients may supposedly be associated with combined hormonal and metabolic disorders even if they were not yet clinically diagnosed. Upon becoming familiar with the cancer risk of combined insulin resistance and estrogen deficiency even in subclinical cases, there would be plenty of possibilities for prevention of malignant tumors in endangered patients.

References

[1] Apridonidze T, Essah PA, Iuorno MJ, et al: Prevalence and characteristics of the metabolic syndrome in women with polycystic ovary syndrome. *J. Clin. Endocrinol. Metab.* 90:1929-1935, 2005

[2] Attia GR, Rainey WE, Carr BR: Metformin directly inhibits androgen production in human thecal cells. *Fertil. Steril.* 76:517-524, 2001

[3] Augustin LSA, Gallus S, Franceschi S, Negri E, Jenkins D, Kendall CWC, dal Maso L, Talamini R, La Vecchia C: Glycemic index and load and risk of upper aero-digestive tract neoplasms. *Cancer Causes and Control* 14:657-662, 2003

[4] Baghaei F, Rosmond R, Westberg L, Hellstrand M, Eriksson E, Holm G, Bjorntorp P: The CYP19 gene and association with a androgens and abdominal obesity in premenopausal women. *Obesity Res.* 11:578-585, 2003

[5] Barros RPA, Machado UF, Gustafsson JA: Estrogen receptors: new players in diabetes mellitus. *Trends Molecular Med.* 9:425-431, 2006

[6] Berrino F, Muti P, Micheli A, Bolelli G, Krogh V, Sciajno R, et al: Serum sex hormon levels after menopause and subsequent breast cancer. *J. Natl. Cancer Inst.* 88:291-296, 1996

[7] Birdsall MA, Farquhar CM, White HD: Association between polycystic ovaries and extent of coronary artery disease in women having cardiac catheterization. *Ann. Intern. Med.* 126:32-35, 1997

[8] Björntorp P: The regulation of adipose tissue distribution in humans. *Int. J. Obes. Relat. Metab. Disord.* 20:291-302, 1996

[9] Bloomgarden ZT: Second World Congress on the Insulin Resistance Syndrome: Mediators, pediatric insulin resistance, the polycystic ovary syndrome, and malignancy. *Diabetes Care* 28:1821-1830, 2005

[10] Bonithon-Kopp C, Scarabin PY, Darne B, Malmejac A, Guize L: Menopause related changes in lipoproteins and some other cardiovascular risk factors. *Int. J. Epidemiol.* 19:42-48, 1990

[11] Bosetti C, Negri E, Franceschi S, Pelucchi C, Talamini R, Montella M, Conti E, La Vecchia C: Diet and ovarian cancer risk: a case-control study in Italy. *Int. J. Cancer* 93:911-915, 2001

[12] Bruning PF, Bonfrer JM, van Noord PA, et al: Insulin resistance and breast cancer risk. *Int. J. Cancer* 52:511-516, 1992

[13] Bryzgalova G, et al: Evidence that oestrogen receptor-alpha plays an important role in the regulation of glucose homeostasis in mice: insulin sensitivity in the liver. *Diabetologia* 49:588-597, 2006

[14] Campbell SE, Febbraio MA: Effect of the ovarian hormones on GLUT4 expression and contraction-stimulated glucose uptake. *Am. J. Physiol. Endocrinol. Metab.* 282:E1139-E1146, 2002

[15] Cara JF, Rosenfield RL: Insulin-like growth factor I and insulin potentiate luteinizing hormone induced androgen synthesis by rat ovarian thecal-interstitial cells. *Endrocrinology* 123:733-739, 1988

[16] Cara JF, Fan J, Azzarello J, Rosenfield RL: Insulin-like growth factor-I enhances luteinizing hormone binding to rat ovarian theca-interstitial cells. *J. Clin. Invest.* 86:560-565, 1990

[17] Carmina E, Lobo RA: Polycystic ovaries in hirsute women with normal menses. *Am. J. Med*: 111:602-606, 2001

[18] Cauley JA, Lucas FL, Kuller LH, Stone K, Browner W, Cummongs SR: Elevated serum estradiol and testosterone concentrations are associated with a high risk for breast cancer. Study of Osteoporotic Fractures Research Group. *Ann. Intern. Med.* 130:270-277, 1999

[19] Cheng CM et al: Estrogen augments glucose transporter and IGF1 expression in primate cerebral cortex. *FASEB J.* 15:907-915, 2001

[20] Cohen JC, Hickman R: Insulin resistance and diminished glucose tolerance in powerlifters ingesting anabolic steroids. *J. Clin. Endocrinol. Metab.* 64:960-963, 1987

[21] Conn JJ, Jacobs HS, Conway GS: The prevalence of polycystic ovaries in women with type-2 diabetes mellitus. *Clin. Endocrinol.* (Oxf) 52:81-86, 2000

[22] Choi SB, Jang JS, Park S: Estrogen and exercise may enhance β-cell function and mass via insulin receptor substrate 2 induction in ovarectomized diabetic rats. *Endocrinology* 146:4786-4794, 2005

[23] Croston GE, Milan LB, Marschke KB, Reichman M, Briggs MR: Androgen receptor-mediated antagonism of estrogen-dependent low density lipoprotein receptor transcription in cultured hepatocytes. *Endocrinology* 138:3779-3786, 1997

[24] Dahlgren E, Johansson S, Lindstedt G, et al: Women with polycystic ovary syndrome wedge resected in 1956 to 1975: a long-term follow-up focusing on natural history and circulating hormones. *Fertil Steril.* 57:505-513, 1992

[25] Dietrich T, Reichart PA, Scheifele C: Clinical risk factors of oral leukoplakia in a representative sample of the US population *Oral Oncol.* 40: 158-163, 2004

[26] Dikshit RP, Ramadas K, Hashibe M, Thomas G, Somanathan T, Sankaranarayanan R: Association between diabetes mellitus and pre-malignant oral diseases: a cross sectional study in Kerala, India. *Int. J. Cancer* 118:453-457, 2006

[27] Distefano E, Marino M, Gillette JA, Hanstein B, Pallottini V, Bruninng J, Krone W, Trentalance A: Role of tyrosine kinase signaling in estrogen induced LDL receptor gene expression in HepG2 cells. *Biochem. Biophys. Acta* 1580:145-149, 2002

[28] Ehrmann DA, Barnes RB, Rosenfield RL, et al: Prevalence of impaired glucose tolerance and diabetes in women with polycystic ovary syndrome. *Diabetes Care* 22:141-146, 1999

[29] Elting MW, Dorsen TJM, Bezemer PD, et al: Prevalence of diabetes mellitus, hypertension and cardiac complaints in a follow-up study of a Dutch PCOS population. *Hum. Reprod.* 16:556-560, 2001

[30] Endogenous Hormones and Breast cancer Collaborative Group. Endogenous sex hormones and breast cancer in postmenopausal women: reanalysis of nine prospective studies. *J. Natl. Cancer Inst.* 94:606-616, 2002

[31] Faustini-Fustini M, Rochira V, Carani C: Oestrogen deficiency in men: where are we today? *Eur. J. Endocrinol.* 140: 111-129, 1999

[32] Ford ES, Giles WH, Mokdad AH: Increasing prevalence of the metabolic syndrome among U.S. adults. *Diabetes Care* 27: 2444-2449, 2004

[33] Fujimoto WY, Bergstrom RW, Boyko EJ, Kinyoun JL, Leonetti DL, Newell-Morris LL, Robinson LR, Shuman WP, Stolov WC, Tsunehara CH, Wahl PW: Diabetes and diabetes risk factors in second- and third-generation Japanese Americans in Seattle, Washington. *Diabetes Res. Clin. Pract.* 24(Suppl):S43-52, 1994

[34] Gadducci A, Gargini A, Palla E, Fanucchi A, Genazzani AR: Polycystic ovary syndrome and gynecological cancers: is there a link? *Gynecol. Endocrinol.* 20:200-208, 2005

[35] Glueck CJ, Papanna R, Wang P, Goldenberg N, Sieve-Smith L: Incidence and treatment of metabolic syndrome in newly referred women with confirmed polycystic ovarian syndrome. *Metabolism* 52:908-915, 2003

[36] Godsland IF, Walton C, Stevenson JC: Impact of menopause on metabolism. In: Diamond MP, Naftolin K, Editors, Matebolism in the female life cycle, Ares Seerono Symposia, Rome 171-189, 1993

[37] Godsland IF: Oestrogens and insulin secretion. *Diabetologia* 48:2213-2220, 2005

[38] Gohlke-Barwolf C: Coronary artery disease: is menopause a risk factor? *Basic Res. Cardiol.* 95:177-183, 2000

[39] Gould GW, Holman GD: The glucose transporter family: structure, function and tissue-specific expression. *Biochem. J.* 295:329-341, 1993

[40] Haffner SM, Katz MS, Stern MP, Dunn JF: The relationship of sex hormones of hyperinsulinemia and hyperglycemia. *Metabolism* 37:683-688, 1988

[41] Hamden K, Carreau S, Ellouz F, Masmoudi H, El FA: Protective effect of 17beta-estradiol on oxidative stress and liver dysfunction in aged male rats. *J. Physiol. Biochem.* 63:195-201, 2007

[42] Heine PA, et al: Increased adipose tissue in male and female estrogen receptor-α knockout mice. *Proc. Natl. Acad. Sci. USA* 97:12729-12734, 2000

[43] Hirose K, Toyama T, Iwata H, et al: Insulin, insulin-like growth factor-1 and breast cancer risk in Japanese women. *Asian Pac. J. Cancer Prev.* 4:239-246, 2003

[44] Hjortland MC, McNamara PM, Kannel WB: Some atherogenic concomitants of menopause: The Framingham Study. *Am. J. Epidemiol.* 103:304-311, 1976

[45] Hu G: Gender difference in all-cause and cardiovascular mortality related to hyperglycaemia and newly diagnosed diabetes. *Diabetologia* 46:608-617, 2003

[46] Jensen J, Nilas L, Christiansen C: Influence of menopause on serum lipids and lipoproteins. *Maturitas* 12:321-331, 1990

[47] Jones ME, et al: Aromatase-deficient (ArKO) mice have a phenotype of increased adiposity. *Proc. Natl. Acad. Sci. USA* 97:12735-12740, 2000

[48] Judd HI, Shamonki IM, Frumar AM, Lagasse LD: Origin of serum estradiol in postmenopausal women. *Obstet Gynecol.* 59:680-686, 1982

[49] Kabuto M, Akiba S, Stevens RG, Neriishi K, Land CE: A prospective study of estradiol and breast cancer in Japanese women. *Cancer Epidemiol. Biomarkers Prev.* 9:575-579, 2000

[50] Kasuga M, et al: The structure of insulin receptor and its subunits. Evidence for multiple non reduced forms and a 210,000 possible proreceptor. *J. Biol. Chem.* 257:10392-10399, 1982

[51] Key TJ, Applyby PN, Reeves GK,: Body mass index, serum sex hormones and breast cancer risk in postmenopausal women. *J. Natl. Cancer Inst.* 95: 1218-1226, 2003

[52] King H, Rewers M, WHO Ad Hoc Diabetes Reporting Group: Global estimates for prevalence of diabetes mellitus and impaired glucose tolerance in adults. *Diabetes Care* 21:157-177, 1993

[53] Legro RS, Kunselman AR, Dobson WE, et al: Prevalence and predictors of risk fortype 2 diabetes mellitus and impaired glucose tolerance in polycystic ovary syndrome: a prospective, controlled study in 254 affected women. *J. Clin. Endocrinol. Metab.* 84: 165-169, 1999

[54] Lewy VD, Danadian K, Witchel SF, Arslanian S, : Early metabolic abnormalities in adolescent girls with polycystic ovarian syndrome. *J. Pediatrics* 138:38-44, 2001

[55] Li C, Briggs RM, Ahlborn ET, Kraemer BF, Liu J: Requirement of Sp1 and Estrogen Receptor α Interaction in 17β-Eastradiol-Mediated Transcriptional Activation of the Low Density Lipoprotein Receptor Gene Expression. *Endocrinology* 142:1546-1553, 2001

[56] Lubahn DB, et al: Alteration of reproductive function but not prenatal sexual development after insertional disruption of the mouse estrogen receptor gene. *Proc. Natl. Acad. Sci. USA* 11162-11166, 1993

[57] Lukits J, Remenar E, Raso E, Ladányi A, Kasler M, Timar J: Molecular identification, expression and prognostic role of estrogen- and progesterone receptors in head and neck cancer. *Int. J. Oncol.* 30:155-160, 2007

[58] Maggiolini M, Donze O, Jeannin E, Ando S, Picard D: Adrenal androgens stimulate the proliferation of breast cancer cells as direct activators of estrogen receptor (alpha). *Cancer Res.* 59:4864-4869, 1999

[59] Matthews KA, Wing RR, Kuller LH, Meilahn EN, Plantinga P: Influence of the perimenopause on cardiovascular risk factors and symptoms of middle-aged healthy women. *Arch Intern. Med.* 154:2349-2355, 1994

[60] Mink PJ, Shahar E, Rosamond WD, Alberg AJ, Folsom AR: Serum insulin and glucose levels and breast cancer incidence: the atherosclerosis risk in communities study. *Am. J. Epidemiol.* 156:349-352, 2002

[61] Moghetti P, Castello R, Negri C, et al: Insulin infusion amplifies 17-(alpha)-hydroxy-corticosteroid intermediates response to adrenocorticotropin in hyperandrogenic women: apparent relative impairment of 17,20-lyase activity. *J. Clin. Endocrinol. Metab.* 81:881-886, 1996

[62] Molteni A, Warpeha RL, Brizio-Molteni L, Fors EM: Estradiol receptor-binding protein in head and neck neoplastic and normal tissue. *Arch Surg.* 116:207-210, 1981

[63] Morales AJ, Laughlin GA, Butzow T, et al: Insulin, somatotropic, and luteinizing hormone axes in lean and obese women with polycystic ovary syndrome: common and distinct features. *J. Clin. Endocrinol. Metab.* 81:2854-2864, 1996

[64] Muraki K, Okuya S, Tanizawa Y: Estrogen receptor alpha regulates insulin sensitivity trough IRS-1 thyrosin phosphorylation in mature 3T3-L1 adipocytes. *Endocr. J.* 53:841-851, 2006

[65] Muti P, Quattrin T, Grant BJB, et al: Fasting glucose is a risk factor for breast cancer. *Cancer Epidemiol. Biomark and Prev.* 11:1361-1368, 2002

[66] Naaz A, et al: Effect of ovariectomy on adipose tissue of mice in the absence of receptor α (ERα): a potential role for estrogen receptor β (ERβ). *Horm. Metab. Res.* 34:758-763, 2002

[67] Nagira K, Sasaoka T, Wada T, Fukui K, Ikubo M, Hori S, Tsuneki H, Saito S, Kobayashi M: Altered subcellular distribution of estrogen receptor is implicated in estradiol-induced dual regulation of insulin signaling in 3T3-L1 adipocytes. *Endocrinology* 147:1020-1028, 2006

[68] Nelson VL, Legro RS, Strauss JF III, et al: Augmented androgen production is a stable steroidogenic phenotype of propagated theca cells from polycystic ovaries. *Mol. Endocrinol.* 13:946-957, 1999

[69] Nestler JE, Jakubowicz DJ: Decreases in ovarian cytochrome P450c17 alpha activity and serum free testosterone after reduction of insulin secretion in polycystic ovary syndrome. *N Engl. J. Med.* 335:617-623, 1996

[70] Nestler JE, Jakubowicz DJ, deVargas AF, et al: Insulin stimulates testosterone biosynthesis by human thecal cells from women polycystic ovary syndrome by activating its own receptor and using inositolglycan mediators as the signal transduction system. *J. Clin. Endocrinol. Metab.* 83:2001-2005, 1998

[71] Nestler JE: Obesity, insulin, sex steroids and ovulation. *Int. J. Obesity and Related Metab. Disorders* 24: 571-573, 2000

[72] Onland-Moret NC, Peeters PHM, van der Schouw YT, Grobbee DE, van Gils CH: Alcohol and endogenous sex steroid levels in postmenopausal women: A cross-sectional study. *J. Clin. Endocrinol. Metab.* 90:1414-1419, 2005

[73] Peppard HR, Marfori J, Luorno MJ, Nestler JE: Prevalence of polycystic ovary syndrome among premenopausal women with type 2 diabetes. *Diabetes Care* 24:1050-1052, 2001

[74] Pierpoint T, McKeigue PM, Isaacs AJ, Wild SH, Jacobs HS: Mortality of women with polycystic ovary syndrome at long-term follow-up. *J. Clin. Epidemiol.* 51:581-586, 1998

[75] Pillay OC, Te Fong LF, Crow JC, Benjamin E, Mould T, Atiomo W, Menon PA, Leonard AJ, Hardiman P: The association between polycystic ovaries and endometrial cancer. *Human Reprod.* 21:924-929, 2006

[76] Potischman N, Gail MH, Troisi R, Wacholder S, Hoover RN: Measurement error does not explain the persistence of the body mass index association with endometrial cancer after adjustment for endogenous hormones. *Epidemiology* 10:76-79, 1999

[77] Proudler AJ, Felton CV, Stevenson JC: Aging and the response of plasma insulin, glucose and C-peptide concentrations to intravenous glucose in postmenopausal women. *Clin. Sci.* 83:489-494, 1992

[78] Rapp K, Schroeder J,Klenk J, Ulmer H, Concin H, Diem G, Oberaigner W, Weiland SK: Fasting blood glucose and cancer risk in a cohort of more than 140,000 adults in Austria. *Diabetologia* 49: 945-952, 2006

[79] Rosenbaum D, et al: Insulin resistance in polycystic ovary syndrome: decreased expression of GLUT-4 glucose transporters in adipocytes. *Am. J. Physiol.* 264:197-202, 1993

[80] Sartor BM, Dickey RP: Polycystic ovarian syndrome and the metabolic syndrome. *Am. J. Med.* 330: 336-342, 2005

[81] Schneider JG, Tompkins C, Blumenthal RS, Mora S: The metabolic syndrome in women. *Cardiol. Rev.* 14:286-291, 2006

[82] Secreto G, Zumoff B: Abnormal production of androgens in women with breast cancer. *Anticancer Res.* 14:2113-2117, 1994

[83] Shi J, Simpkins JW: 17β-Estradiol modulation of glucose transporter 1 expression in blood-brian barrier. *Am. J. Physiol.* 272:1016-1022, 1997

[84] Soliman PT, Oh JC, Schmeler KM, Sun CC, Slomovitz BM, Gershenson DM, Burke TW, Lu KH: Risk factors for young premenopausal women with endometrial cancer. *Obstet Gynecol.* 105:575-580, 2005

[85] Solomon CG et al: Long or highly irregular menstrual cycles as a marker for risk of type-2 diabetes mellitus. *JAMA* 286:2421-2426, 2001

[86] Spritzer PM, Morsch DM, Wiltgen D: Polycystic ovary syndrome associated neoplasms. *Arq. Bras. Endocrinol. Metabol.* 49:805-810, 2006

[87] Stattin P, Bjor O, Ferrari P, Lukanova A, Lenner P, Lindahl B, Hallmans G, Kaaks R: Prospective study of hyperglycemia and cancer risk. *Diabetes Care* 30:561-567, 2007

[88] Suba Zs: Gender-related hormonal risk factors for oral cancer. *Pathol Oncol. Res.* 13:195-202, 2007

[89] Sugaya A et al: Expression of glucose transporter 4 mRNA in adipose tissue and skeletal muscle of ovariectomized rats treated with sex steroid hormones. *Life Sci.* 66:641-648, 2000

[90] Talbott E, Guzick D, Clerici A, et al: Coronary heart disease risk factors in women with polycystic ovary syndrome. *Arteroscler. Thromb. Vasc. Biol.* 15:821-826, 1995

[91] Talbott EO, Zborowski JV, Rager JR, Boudreaux MY, Edmundowicz DA, Guzick DS: Evidence for an association between metabolic cardiovascular syndrome and coronary and aortic calcification among women with polycystic ovary syndrome. *J. Clin. Endocrinol. Metab.* 89:5454-5461, 2004

[92] Taylor AE, McCourt B, Martin K, et al: Determinants of abnormal gonadotropin secretion in clinically defined women with PCOS. *J. Clin. Endocrinol. Metab.* 82:2248-2256, 1997

[93] Waldstreicher J, Santoro NF, Hall JE, et al: Hyperfunction of the hypothalamic-pituitary axis in women with polycystic ovarian disease: indirect evidence for partial gonadotroph desensitization. *J. Clin. Endocrinol. Metab.* 66:165-172, 1988

[94] Walsh BW, Schiff I, Rosner B, Greenberg L, Ravinkar V, Sacks FM: Effects of postmenopausal estrogen replacement on the concentrations and metabolism of plasma lipoproteins. *New England J. Med.* 325:1196-1204, 1991

[95] Welch RD, Gorski J: Regulation of glucose transporters by estradiol in the immature rat uterus. *Endocrinology* 140:3602-3608, 1999

[96] Westberg L, Baghaei F, Rosmond R, Hellstrand M, Landén M, Jansson M, Holm G, Björntorp P, Eriksson E: Polymorphisms of the androgen receptor gene and the estrogen receptor-β gene are associated with androgen levels in women. *J. Clin. Endocrinol. Metab.* 86:2562-2568, 2001

[97] Wilson PWE: Does estrogen reduce glycemic levels? *Diabetes Care* 21:1585-1586, 1998

[98] Wu ShI, Chou P, Tsai ShT: The impact of years since menopause on the development of impaired glucose tolerance. *J. Clin. Epidemiol.* 54:117-120, 2001

[99] Zhou L, et al: Action of insulin receptor substrate-3 (IRS-3) and IRS-4 to stimulate translocation of GLUT4 in rat adipose cells. *Mol. Endocrinol.* 13:505-514, 1999

Chapter 8

Hormonal and Metabolic Risk Factors for Oral Cancer among Non-smoker, Non-drinker Women

The Mystery of Smoking Associated Cancers without Smoking

After incursions in the field of insulin resistance, estrogen deficiency and their combinations, let's return to the mystery of non-smoker, non-drinker oral cancer cases.

In the past century oral cancer was regarded as a typically tobacco and alcohol associated tumor of middle-aged and elderly male patients. The excessive smoking and drinking habits of men as compared with women were regarded as plausible explanations to the conspicuously high male to female incidence ratio of oral cancer (see Chapter 1). Krolls and coworkers in 1976 established a male to female ratio of 13.1 in their study on oral cancer cases [21], whereas, nowadays this ratio decreased to near 2:1 in the United States [8].

Fifty years ago a comprehensive study on oral cancer patients in the United States established that 97% of the male patients were or had been smokers [50]. In the early 80s a decreasing ratio of smokers among male oral cancer cases resulted in a 76% prevalence of smokers [35]. In Hungary, the steeply increasing morbidity and mortality rates for oral cancer are associated with decreasing ratio of smokers (see Chapter 1).

Strict restriction of smoking in some economically developed countries resulted in a transitory decrease in oral cancer incidence at the end of the past century. However, recently, yet unknown risk factors and a new wave of increased prevalence of oral cancer have arisen (see Chapter 1).

Non-smoker oral cancer cases have always occurred in many populations, and it was a challenge to explain the origin of these malignancies. For a long time, an increased prevalence of elderly female patients among non-smoker, non-drinker oral cancer cases have been observed without rational explanation (see Chapter 1 and 5).

A systemic risk factor for oral cancer independent of tobacco was first suggested about 50 years ago. In anemic, middle aged and elderly women, atrophy of the oral and upper gastrointestinal mucosa was found to be associated with high risk for oral cancer [45,50].

Joynson and coworkers demonstrated impairment of cell-mediated immunity in iron-deficient patients, which was regarded as player in the pathogenesis of chronic infections and malignant diseases [17]. Iron-deficiency anemia in animal experiments resulted in atrophy, reduced maturation and disturbed keratinisation in the oral epithelium suggesting increased susceptibility to chemical carcinogens [34].

Clinical epidemiological studies also supported the correlation between sideropenia of elderly females and oral cancer risk [4,35], however, a direct, causal association between these two alterations was not justified. High incidence of oral cancer among non-smoker, non-drinker elderly females remained an unanswered question.

Diet and nutritional factors also begin to emerge in the etiology of oral and pharyngeal cancers in the early 80s [49]. Recently, authors from Italy and Switzerland published data that a Mediterranean diet rich in fish, vegetables and fruits seems to be beneficial not only against oropharyngeal cancers but against tumors at other sites (see Chapter 2). These findings suggest that a healthy diet may exert its beneficial effects not only in the oral cavity but also by favorable modulation of the metabolic processes. Moreover, Mediterranean diet may moderate even the carcinogenic effects of tobacco and alcohol in the oral region (see Chapter 2). Unfortunately, these literary data do affect neither the gender-related differences of oral cancer prevalence nor the accumulation of non-smoker, elderly women among oral cancer cases.

Controversies in global trends of oral cancer epidemiology in the last decades have raised many questions to be answered. Nowadays, the earlier markedly high male to female ratio of oral cancer incidence has shown a rapidly decreasing tendency in many countries. The increasing prevalence of women among oral cancer cases as compared with men has been regarded simply as a result of their similarly excessive smoking habits. However, a shocking feature of oral cancer epidemiology today is the increasing prevalence of non-smoker, non-drinker cases, especially among older female patients (see Chapter 1).

The increasing incidence rate of oral cancer among very young cases less than 30 years old of age is also alarming. Epidemiology of oral cancer in the young conspicuously differs from that of older patients concerning the near equal or even inverse male to female incidence ratio of the disease. Primacy of lingual location in young oral cancer cases is also contradictory to the high predominance of sublingual cancers among older patients. Nevertheless, smoking and excessive alcohol intake as risk factors may be completely excluded in oral cancer cases under 30 years of age as there is not enough time for carcinogen-induced cancer to develop from its initiation (see Chapter 1).

The majority of contradictory epidemiological changes in oral cancer incidence are associated with gender-related differences. Moreover, smoking and drinking habits may usually not explain the increasing number of controversial changes in oral cancer epidemiology. Consequently, we are on the route to reject smoking and drinking as determinant risk factors for oral cancer.

Our working group first published the significant epidemiological associations between type-2 diabetes and oral cancer on a pooled, male-female population of patients in Hungary (see Chapter 3). Since then these correlations have been strengthened by several studies. Later, separated investigations of male and female patients with oral cancer revealed conspicuous gender related epidemiological differences. A preferential risk of elevated fasting glucose and long lasting estrogen deficiency for oral cancer was established among predominantly postmenopausal female patients (see Chapter 5).

A new Hungarian case-control study was performed on non-smoker, non-drinker female oral cancer cases to answer the following questions:

1. Which are the possible risk factors for oral cancer among non-smoker, non-drinker women?
2. Why does oral cancer exhibit a decreasing trend of the earlier very high male to female ratio?
3. What is the explanation to the continuously increasing prevalence of non-smoker, non-drinker cases among oral cancer patients?
4. How can the equalization trend of male to female ratio of oral cancer cases in the young under 30 years of age be explained?

Case-control Study of Non-smoker, Non-drinker Women with Oral Cancer in Hungary

At the Department of Oral and Maxillofacial Surgery 250 female cases with oral cancer were admitted between 1 January 2003 and 31 December 2007. As controls, 250 tumor-free women were selected from our outpatient cases with dental diseases. For all cancer cases age-matched controls within half year were selected. Data of oral cancer cases and their controls were collected via case reports and questionnaires. Smoker and non-smoker, non-drinker (NSND) patient groups were separately studied both among oral cancer cases and controls. In this study on female oral cancer patients 49.6% were smokers, whereas 50.4% were NSND cases.

Age of patients. The mean age of women with oral cancer was 63.2 years and that of controls was 63.5 years. The mean age of smokers among women with oral cancer was significantly lower (59.4 yrs) as compared with that of NSND oral cancer cases (66.1 yrs). Age distribution among smoker and non-smoker women with oral cancer was quite different. Among smoker oral cancer patients, the vast majority of cases (68.2%) were between 46 and 64 years of age, whereas among NSND oral cancer women a predominance of cases over 65 years of age (64.6%) was observed. Consequently, among smoker women with oral cancer, not only the mean age was markedly lower as compared with non-smokers, but also a significant accumulation of middle-aged cases was conspicuous as compared with the predominantly elderly non-smoker oral cancer cases.

Tumor locations. Among women with oral cancer, gingival cancer was the most common tumor location. Among *smoker oral cancer cases* sublingual region was the most common tumor site (41.8%) followed in decreasing order by the gingiva (24.5%), the tongue (19.4%) and other rare locations. However, among *NSND women with oral cancer* the most common tumor site was the gingiva (29.4%), followed by the tongue (17.6%), the sublingual region (14.1%) and other rare locations. Based on these data, a close association of exogenous noxae and sublingual tumor location may be justified. However, in NSND cases the primacy of gingival cancer seems to be similar to the high rate of gingival tumors among all oral cancer cases.

Metabolic factors. Rates of obesity and elevated fasting glucose level (EFG) were established among oral cancer cases and controls (Table 8.1). Obesity was registered at admission if the patient exhibited a body mass index (BMI) above 30kg/m^2. Weight loss in the history of patients was disregarded, as these anamnestic data were not controllable. EFG was established if the fasting glucose level was repeatedly equal or above 5.5 mmol/l.

The *rate of obesity* among all women with oral cancer was 25.5%, whereas in the tumor-free control group it was moderately lower: 19.6%. Obesity rate among smoker oral cancer cases was slightly lower (15.9%) as compared with smoker control women (17.1%). However, among NSND oral cancer cases obesity rate was significantly higher (33.4%) than among non-smoker control cases (21.1%). These data reveal that obesity is a high risk factor for oral cancer among NSND women in contrast with smoker cases.

The *rate of elevated fasting glucose* was significantly higher in the group of oral cancer cases (57.9%) as compared with the tumor-free controls (41.5). The elevated fasting glucose rate among smoker oral cancer cases was moderately higher (55.1%) as compared with their smoker controls (43.5%). However, among NDNA oral cancer cases the rate of elevated fasting glucose was significantly higher (60.4%) as compared with their NDNA controls (39.2%). Smoker control cases were markedly younger as compared with NSND controls as they were properly matched to the oral cancer group, however, they exhibited higher rate of EFG as compared with NSND controls. Elevated fasting glucose proved to be a much higher risk factor for oral cancer among NSND cases than among smoker cases.

Reproductive factors (Table 8.2). The rate of pre- and postmenopausal cases among women with oral cancer was compared with that of their age matched controls. The rate of long or irregular menstrual cycles and infertility suggesting hormonal disorders and mean age at menopause were compared between smoker and NDNA oral cancer groups and their controls. Rates of early and late menopause as well as hysterectomy among patients with oral cancer and their controls were also registered. Mean time interval between menopause and oral cancer diagnosis (M-OC) were calculated in the smoker and NSND groups with oral cancer.

The *rate of postmenopausal cases* was 94.9% among all patients with oral cancer, whereas among age-matched control females it was significantly lower (80.2%). Among smoker cases with oral cancer the rate of premenopausal state was as low as 2.6%, whereas 7.8% of NSND patients with oral cancer were premenopausal. Among control women 16.5% of smokers were premenopausal, however in the NSND group the rate of premenopausal cases was significantly higher; 23.2%.

Table 8.1. Rate of obesity and elevated fasting glucose (EFG) among patients with oral cancer and their controls

Metabolic disorders	Oral Cancer			Control		
	All	Smoker	NSND	All	Smoker	NSND
Obesity	25.5%	15.9%	33.4%	19.6%	17.1%	21.1%
EFG	57.9%	55.1%	60.4%	41.5%	43.5%	39.2%

Table 8.2. History of reproductive data of females with oral cancer and their controls

Reproductive data	Oral Cancer			Control		
	All	Smoker	NSND	All	Smoker	NSND
Postmenopausal cases (%)	94.9%	97.4%	92.2%	80.2%	83.5%	76.8%
Hormonal disorders (%)	15.2%	16.5%	14.0%	10.6%	13.5%	8.9%
Mean age of menopause (yrs)	46.7	45.1	48.4	50.6	48.1	51.9
Early menopause (<45yrs) (%)	24.6%	27.1%	21.7%	16.4%	19.8%	13.8%
Late menopause (>50yrs) (%)	13.0%	8.8%	17.1%	25.3%	21.9%	28.5%
Hysterectomy cases (%)	29.3%	30.8%	28.5%	17.6%	19.5%	15.1%
Mean M-OC interval (yrs)	17.5	14.2	21.4	-	-	-

Rate of hormonal disorders in the patients' history was not significantly higher in the oral cancer group as compared with the control cases (15.2% and 10.6%, respectively). Among smoker oral cancer cases the rate of hormonal disorders was moderately higher (16.5%) as compared with their non-smoker controls (13.5%). In the NSND group with oral cancer, the rate of hormonal disorders was significantly higher (14.0%) than that of their non-smoker controls (8.9%).

Mean age at menopause among the oral cancer cases was 46.7 years, whereas among the controls it was 50.6 years. Mean age at menopause was lower among smoker oral cancer cases (45.1 years) as compared with NSND cases (48.4). In the tumor-free control group mean age at menopause was also lower among smokers (48.1 years) as compared with non-smokers (51.9 years).

The *rate of early menopause* (before 45 yrs) among all oral cancer cases was 24.6%, whereas in the tumor-free control group it was significantly lower: 16.4%. Rate of early menopause in the smoker subgroup of oral cancer cases was 27.1%, whereas in their NSND subgroup it was 21.7%. In the control group this rate was significantly lower both in the smoker and non-smoker subgroups (19.8% and 13.8%, respectively).

The *rate of late menopause* (after 50 yrs) was significantly lower in the oral cancer group (13%) as compared with the control group (25.3%). Among smoker women with oral cancer this rate was much lower (8,8%), whereas among NSND oral cancer cases 17.1%. Among controls the rate of late menopause was significantly higher: 28.5% in the NDNA control group and 21.9% in the smoker control group.

Rates of hysterectomy among oral cancer cases and their controls showed significant differences (29.3% and 17.6% respectively). Among smoker oral cancer cases 30.8% had hysterectomy in their history, while among NSND cases with oral cancer the rate of hysterectomy was lower; 28.5%. Among the smoker control cases the rate of hysterectomy was higher (19.5) than among non-smokers (15.1). In the control group of women the rate of hysterectomy was significantly lower both among smokers and non-smokers.

Mean M-OC time interval was 17.5 years in the pooled oral cancer group of women. Among smoker oral cancer cases the M-OC interval was significantly shorter (14.2 yrs) as compared with that of NSND cases (21.4 yrs). Among the smoker women with oral cancer, the mean M-OC time interval was shorter in the majority of cases (69.1%) as compared with that of all female patients. In contrast, in the NSND group with oral cancer the rate of short M-OC time interval was significantly lower (35.5%).

Hypothyroidism. Rates of earlier diagnosed and treated thyroid hormone deficiency caused by thyroiditis or strumectomy were registered in the oral cancer and control groups. Serum thyroid hormone and TSH levels were not available.

In the pooled oral cancer group the rate of overt hypothyroidism was 5.6%, whereas among all control cases it was 2.4% ($p<0.05$). Separate analysis of the rate of hypothyroidism in the smoker and NSND groups of oral cancer cases revealed significant differences. The rate of hypothyroidism was 2.8% among the smoker oral cancer cases and significantly higher; 8.3% in the NSND group with oral cancer. Among the controls, the rate of hypothyroidism was within the normal range of population data; 2.9% in the group of smokers and 2.0% among NSND cases.

Risk factors for oral cancer among premenopausal patients. In this study, only 8 premenopausal cases were found in the group of women with oral cancer, 6 in the NSND and 2 in the smoker group.

Out of the 8 premenopausal NSND cases 2 women exhibited diagnosed polycystic ovarium syndrome. In 2 cases long lasting type-2 diabetes and in 2 cases infertility and test tube baby program was found in the history. In one case premenopausal hypothyroidism was diagnosed. In 1 of premenopausal, non-smoker oral cancer cases no clinically diagnosed systemic risk factor for oral cancer was found.

Nevertheless, in this study, laboratory findings justifying subclinical hyperinsulinemia, estrogen deficiency or hypothyroidism were not available. Data of the patients were based on clinical case reports and questionnaires. Subclinical metabolic and hormonal disorders without exhibition of overt diseases could also occur among the oral cancer cases and controls.

Risk Factors for Oral Cancer other than Tobacco and Alcohol

The presented results related to non-smoker, non-drinker women revealed that the postmenopausal state and some disorders associated with estrogen loss might be regarded as risk factors for oral cancer.

Obesity was not a cancer risk factor among pooled oral cancer cases; in contrast, among NSND women it proved to be significant risk for oral cancer. Elevated fasting glucose level, reflecting any stage of insulin resistance proved to be stronger risk for oral cancer in NSND women than in smoker cases. Furthermore, overt hypothyroidism in the history of NSND women showed significant correlation with their oral cancer risk.

These results do not oppose to the carcinogenic capacity of smoking and excessive alcohol use but rather prove that they do not have exclusive role in oral carcinogenesis.

Till now, the local intraoral effects of tobacco and alcohol were regarded as the only aspects of their carcinogenic capacity. Justification of the causal role of insulin resistance and estrogen deficiency in oral cancer risk rather suggests that tobacco and alcohol are only two of many factors, which may disadvantageously influence the hormonal and metabolic equilibrium of the patients (see Chapters 2 and 5).

These bad habits have primary local carcinogenic effects on the oral mucosa, which have been a deceiving feature of their carcinogenic capacity for a long time. This evident, contact impact of smoking and alcohol derivatives disguised the second, more effective step of their carcinogenicity, the long lasting metabolic and hormonal disorders, which return again to the oral cavity as a systemic factor.

Newly recognized cancer risk factors, such as fat-rich diet, physical inactivity, obesity and inherited inclination to type-2 diabetes may primarily provoke insulin resistance. The associated estrogen deficiency in women will be a further step on the route leading to cancer initiation and promotion. Tobacco and excessive alcohol intake may work similarly as they have decreasing effect on insulin sensitivity and estrogen level (see Chapter 2).

However, inherited or acquired pathologic states may induce primarily estrogen deficiency. This alteration may be caused by defect of aromatase activity, ovarian insufficiency, hysterectomy, repeated abortions and menopause with disturbed adaptation. These estrogen deficient states do induce parallel insulin resistance, which may also lead to cancer initiation (see Chapter 7).

Moderate alcohol consumption is an important factor to preserve the metabolic and hormonal equilibrium in postmenopausal cases. Regular, moderate alcohol intake shows beneficial effect on cardiovascular and all cause mortality of elderly women, which may be attributed to the increased insulin sensitivity and elevated estrogen level (see Chapter 2). In the presented study, complete abstinence of middle aged or elderly women among NSND cases may have a role in their high ratio of obesity and elevated fasting glucose, which are proven risk factors for cancer initiation (see Chapter 2).

Smoking has well known correlations with insulin resistance (see Chapter 2), however, associations of hypothyroidism with smoking habits seem to be controversial. Recently, lower prevalence of overt hypothyroidism was observed among current smokers as compared with non-smokers [3]. Nevertheless, exhibition of symptoms in hypothyroidism strongly depends on the age of patients, the younger the patient the stronger the complaints caused by hypothyroidism. On the contrary, among elderly cases hypothyroidism is frequently overlooked, as laboratory findings are not associated with diagnosable clinical symptoms [16]. Consequently, only strictly age-adjusted studies may authentically reflect the correlation between tobacco use and overt hypothyroidism.

A novel hypothesis based on the results of this study is hypothyroidism as a risk factor for oral cancer. Nevertheless, among our patients with oral cancer, overt hypothyroidism is only a tip of the iceberg among many subclinical cases, as symptom-free mild hypothyroidism is especially frequent among middle aged and older women [14].

Questions to be Answered in Oral Cancer Epidemiology

The first question was the nature of possible risk factors for oral cancer in non-smoker, non-drinker cases.

Summarizing the effects of different exogenous and systemic cancer risk factors, it can be established that recognition of the carcinogenic impact of insulin resistance, estrogen deficiency and hypothyroidism revealed a common pathway through which many harmful factors may exert their carcinogenic capacity.

The second question to be answered was the cause of the global, increasing ratio of female cases among oral cancer patients and the continuous decrease of the earlier conspicuously high male to female ratio of oral cancer incidence.

Glucose intolerance and type-2 diabetes have increasing prevalence all over the world, seeming to be an oral cancer risk preferentially among postmenopausal women. Insulin resistance combined with estrogen deficiency means a high risk factor for oral cancer among women but lower among men (see Chapter 5). Though prevalence of insulin resistance exhibits also an increasing trend among male populations, they are not so highly endangered by metabolic cancer initiation.

The third question was the cause of the increasing prevalence of non-smoker, non-drinker cases among oral cancer patients.

Decreased population of smokers, especially in the economically developed countries helped to emerge further, earlier hidden systemic cancer risk factors, such as insulin resistance and estrogen deficiency (see Chapter 1). The present study justified that less than half of the women with oral cancer were never smokers or drinkers, and their vast majority exhibited chronic hormonal and metabolic disturbances, which may be regarded as risk factors for oral cancer. These epidemiological features supply additional data to the increasing rate of oral cancer morbidity without smoking.

The fourth problem is the low, equalized or even inverse male to female ratio among very young oral cancer cases (<30 yrs), which highly differs from the high male to female ratio of middle aged or elderly patients.

This may also be explained by the higher cancer risk of systemic hormonal disorders for women as compared with men. Ovarian insufficiency and glucose intolerance may develop insidiously in young girls even in puberty (see Chapter 6). Higher rate of estrogen deficiency and parallel insulin resistance in girls and higher sensitivity of their organs for hormonal disorders as compared with boys may result in excess of female oral cancer cases.

The primacy of tongue location of intraoral cancers in both genders of the young may be hard to explain. In older patients with oral cancer the typical sublingual tumor location can be justified by some exogenous noxae, which are solved in the saliva in the horseshoe between the mandible and tongue (see Chapter 1). However, in oral cancer of the young perhaps the highest frequency of mechanical injuries on the lateral border of the tongue may complete the carcinogenic capacity of mild or moderate hormonal and metabolic disorders.

Recently, correlations among smoking, alcohol consumption and the associated metabolic and hormonal disorders have been increasingly studied. Beneficial, anticancer effects of Mediterranean diet, red wine and hormone replacement therapy were reported and these associations were independent of smoking status of the patients (see Chapter 2 and 4). The presented systemic cancer risk factors for non-smoker, non-drinker women might shed a beam of light on the mystery of smoking associated cancers without smoking.

Metabolic and Hormonal Associations of Hypothyroidism

Thyroid hormone deficiency causes hypothyroidism, which has an increased prevalence in women, especially in older age. Overt diseases are relatively rare, with a 2-3% incidence rate among women and 0.5-1.0% among men. In young adults, weakness, fatigue, peripheral myxedema, weight gain, cold intolerance and increased rate of cardiovascular events are the predominant features [38]. On the contrary, in elderly patients low thyroid hormone and elevated thyroid-stimulating hormone (TSH) levels are rarely associated with clinical symptoms.

Subclinical hypothyroidism is characterized by normal serum free thyroxin and elevated serum TSH concentrations [38]. Subclinical hypothyroidism is a prevalent condition among the adult population, however it is frequently overlooked. Recently, subclinical, undiagnosed hypothyroidism and its correlations with other hormonal and metabolic alterations have been thoroughly studied.

Thyroid hormones are crucial regulators of lipid metabolism [32]. Hypothyroidism even in subclinical forms has close associations with dyslipidemia [44]. Subclinical hypothyroidism is closely associated with low-grade inflammation, increased serum triglyceride, lipoprotein and cholesterol levels [15,20,22,29].

Literary data support the beneficial effect of thyroid hormone administration on disturbed lipid metabolism and cardiovascular risk in patients with subclinical hypothyroidism [26,33]. L-thyroxine therapy regulates the decreased HDL cholesterol level in patients with hypothyroidism. Hormonal treatment of hypothyroidism is advantageous in cases of metabolic disorders and hyperinsulinemia [43].

There are close correlations between hypothyroidism and insulin resistance. Thyroid functions affect all parameters of the metabolic syndrome including HDL cholesterol level, triglycerides, blood pressure and plasma glucose level [18,19,42]. Increased prevalence of subclinical hypothyroidism could be observed among patients with metabolic syndrome, especially in females [42]. Rates of diabetes mellitus, glucose intolerance and obesity are also increased among patients with hypothyroidism [43]. These data support the important role of diagnosis and treatment of hypothyroidism in the metabolic control of insulin resistance.

Hypothyroidism may worsen many risk factors for cardiovascular disease, including hypertension, abnormal endothelial function elevate low-density and decrease high-density lipoprotein cholesterol concentrations [6,11,12,30,44]. In epidemiological studies, subclinical hypothyroidism was associated with atherosclerosis [5] and with increased risk for ischemic heart disease [2,25] and negatively affected cardiovascular and all-cause mortality [16,31]. L-thyroxin treatment has beneficial improvement on cardiovascular risk factors and quality of life in cases with subclinical hypothyroidism [33].

Myxedema of overt hypothyroidism was associated with increased peripheral vascular resistance and hypercholesterolemia as well, which are risk factors for ischemic cardiovascular disease [27]. Low triiodothyronin level was a significant predictor of l-year mortality among patients admitted for acute stroke [1].

Infertility and ovulation disorders might also be associated with subclinical thyroid dysfunction [13]. Evaluation of thyroid gland function seems to be an indispensable part of investigation procedure in infertile women [28].

Till now, epidemiological associations of hypothyroidism with oral cancer risk have not been investigated. However, close correlation of hypothyroidism with insulin resistant and estrogen deficient states may probably mean a connection between thyroid hormone deficiency and cancer. Confirmation of these findings requires further investigations.

Similar Mechanisms of Genomic and Nongenomic Actions of Thyroid and Steroid Hormones

Thyroid and steroid hormones, despite their distinct structures and biologic effects, have surprising similarities in their genomic and non-genomic actions [10,51]. They are thought primarily to act via binding to hormone-specific nuclear receptor superfamily members, and the nuclear ligand-receptor complexes then initiate transcriptional activity [36,41]. Moreover, both steroids and thyroid hormones have also non-genomic actions through their membrane-associated receptor system [10].

Thyroid hormones may exert their genomic actions via diffusion across the plasma membrane and interaction with intranuclear receptors. Liganded receptors exert their major action at the nuclear transcription level by regulating the level of mRNAs of specific genes [7]. Thyroid receptors have important action on gene activation and gene silencing [41]. They can bind to DNA even in the absence of ligand. Although in most cases they cannot activate target genes in such a way, they are not neutral in regulating target gene expression. In the absence of hormones, they frequently abrogate the basal promoter activity. These gene-silencing mechanisms may have pivotal significance in the pathology of hypothyroidism.

Thyroid receptors are regulators of the intermediary metabolism and can up-regulate enzymes and cytochromes involved in mitochondrial function [48] and have associations with lipid peroxidation [40]. Furthermore, they are involved in glucose transport and glucose metabolism [46] and have close correlations with gene regulatory activities of dietary fat, like polyunsaturated fatty acids (PUFAs) [18,39,47]. Thorough studies on correlations between lipid metabolism, thyroid hormone signals and gene regulation justify the metabolic and cell proliferation disorders in hypothyroidism.

Similarly to steroid hormones, thyroid hormones may exert also non-genomic or extranuclear actions via membrane-associated receptors [10]. Thyroid hormones appear to interact with specific cell surface G protein coupled receptors and to activate signal-transducing kinases such as those involved in the mitogen-activated protein kinase (MAPK) pathway [23,37]. In cultured cells thyroid hormone potentiates the action of epidermal growth factor [24]. These non-genomic mechanisms of thyroid hormone receptors may modulate the cellular activities of cytokines and growth factors and their action may be severely altered by thyroid hormone deficiency.

There are similar interfaces of non-genomic and genomic actions of thyroid hormones as compared with estrogens. Thyroid hormones are able to promote serine phosphorylation of the nuclear thyroid receptors also by non-genomic mechanism and by such phosphorylation the transcriptional activity of the nuclear receptor proteins may be altered [9,37].

Similarities of genomic and non-genomic actions of thyroid and steroid hormones suggest that these hormones may have similar roles in the defense mechanisms against cancer initiation. Presumably these hormone families have thorough interplays, and decreased hormonal signal of each one may provoke contraregulatory effects of the other one. The above mentioned literary data suggest that estrogen and thyroid hormone deficiency together, even in subclinical form, may exert severe disturbances in the gene regulation level. This may be associated with increased risk for insulin resistance, type-2 diabetes and infertility in women as well as for cancer.

References

[1] Alevizaki M, Synetou M, Xynos K, Pappa T, Vemmos KN: Low triiodothyronine: a strong predictor of outcome in acute stroke patients. *European Journal of Clinical Investigation* 37:651-657, 2007

[2] Althaus BU, Staub J-J, Ryff-De Léche A, Oberhänsli A, and Stähelin HB: LDL/HDL-changes in subclinical hypothyroidism: possible risk factors for coronary heart disease. *Clinical Endocrinology* 28:157-163, 1988

[3] Asvold BO, Bjoro T, Nilsen TI, Vatten LJ: Tobacco smoking and thyroid function: a population-based study. *Archives of Internal Medicine* 167:1428-1432, 2007

[4] Binnie WH, Rankin KV, Mackenzie IC: Etiology of oral squamous cell carcinoma. *J. Oral Path* 12:11-29, 1983

[5] Cappola AR, Ladenson PW: Hypotyroidism and atherosclerosis. *Journal of Clinical Endocrinology and Metabolism* 88:2438-2444, 2003

[6] Caron P, Calazel C, Parra HJ, Hoff M, and Louvet JP: Decreased HDL cholesterol in subclinical hypothyreoidism: the effect of L-thyroxine therapy. *Clinical Endocrinology* 33:519-523, 1990

[7] Chin WW, Yen PM: Molecular mechanisms of nuclear thyroid hormone action. In: Braverman LE. Contemporary endocrinology: Diseases of the thyroid. Humana Press, Totowa, 1997, p.1.

[8] Clayman L: Oral cancer. A practical guide to understanding oral cancer. ELLM Press, 2002

[9] Davis PJ, Shih A, Lin H-Y, Martino LJ, Davis FB: Thyroxine promotes association of mitogen-activated protein kinase and nuclear thyroid hormone receptor (TR) and causes serine phosphorylation of TR. J. *Biol. Chem.* 275:38032-38039, 2000

[10] Davis PJ, Tillmann HC, Davis FB, Wehling M: Comparison of the mechanisms of nongenomic actions of thyroid hormone and steroid hormones. *Journal of Endocrinological Investigation* 25:377-388, 2002

[11] Duntas LH, Wartofsky L: Cardiovascular risk and subclinical hypothyroidism: focus on lipids and new emerging risk factors. What is the evidence?. *Thyroid* 17:1075-1084, 2007

[12] Duggal J, Singh S, Barsano CP, Arora R: Cardiovascular risk with subclinical hyperthyroidism and hypothyreoidism: pathophysiology and management. *Journal of the CardioMetabolic Syndrome* 2:198-206, 2007

[13] Eldar-Geva T, Shohan M, Rosler A, Margalioth EJ, Livne K, Meirow D: Subclinical hypothyroidism in infertile women: the importance of continuous monitoring and the role of the thyrotropin-releasing hormone stimulation test. *Gynecological Endocrinology* 23:332-337, 2007

[14] Hak AE, Pols HA, Visser TJ, Drexhage HA, Hofman A, and Witteman JC: Subclinical hypothyroidism is an independent risk factor for atheroclerosis and myocardial infarction in elderly women: the Rotterdam study. *Ann. Intern. Med.* 132:270-278, 2000

[15] Hueston WJ, and Pearson WS: Subclinical hypothyroidism and the risk of hypercholesterolemia. *Annals of Family Medicine* 2:351-355, 2004

[16] Imaizumi M, Akahoshi M, Ichimaru S, Nakashima E, Hida A, Soda M, Usa T, Ashizawa K, Yokoyama N, Maeda R, Nagataki S, Eguchi K: Risk for ishemic heart disease and all-cause mortality in subclinical hypothyroidism. *Journal of Clinical Endocrinology and Metabolism* 89:3365-3370, 2004

[17] Joynson DH, Walker DM, Jacobs A, Dolby AE: Defect of cell-mediated immunity in patients with iron-deficiency anemia. *Lancet* 2:1058-1059, 1972

[18] Jump DB, Clarke SD, Thelen A, Liimatta M, Ren B, Badin MV: Dietary fat, genes, and human health. *Advances in Experimental Medicine and Biology* 422:167-176, 1997

[19] Jung CH, Sung KC, Shin HSS, Rhee EJ, Lee WY, Kim BS, Kang JH, Kim H, Kim SW, Lee MH, Park JR, and Kim SW: Thyroid dysfunction and their relation to cardiovascular risk factors such as lipid profile, hsCRP, and waist hip ratio in Korea. *Korean Journal of Internal Medicine* 18:146-153, 2003

[20] Kung AW, Pang RW, Janus ED: Elevated serum lipoprotein in subclinical hypothyroidism. *Clin. Endocrinol.* 43:445-449, 1995

[21] Krolls SO, Hoffman S: Squamous cell carcinoma of the oral soft tissues: a statistical analysis of 14,253 cases by age, sex, and race of patients. *JADA* 92:571-574, 1976

[22] Kvetny J, Heldgaard PE, Bladbjerg EM, and Gram J: Subclinical hypothyroidism is associated with a low-grade inflammation, increased triglyceride levels and predicts cardiovascular disease in males below 50 years. *Clinical Endocrinology* 61:232-238, 2004

[23] Lin H-Y, Davis FB, Gordinier JK, Martino LJ, Davis PJ: Thyroid hormone induces activation of mitogen-activated protein kinase in cultured cells. *Am. J. Physiol.* 276:1014-1024, 1999

[24] Lin HY, Shih A, Davis FB, Davis PJ: Thyroid hormone promotes the phosphorylation of STAT3 and potentiates the action of epidermal growth factor in cultured cells. *Biochem. J.* 338:427-432, 1999

[25] Luboshitzky R, Aviv A, Herer P, Lavie L: Risk factors for cardiovascular disease in women with subclinical hypothyroidism. *Thyroid* 12:421-425, 2002

[26] Miura S, Iitaka M, Yoshimura H, Kitahama S, Fukasawa N, Kawakami Y, Sakurai S, Urabe M, Sakatsume Y, Ito K, Ishii J: Disturbed lipid metabolism in patients with subclinical hypothyroidism: effect of L-thyroxine therapy. *Internal Medicine* 33:413-417, 1994

[27] Mohr-Kahaly S, Kahaly G, Meyer J: Cardiovascular effects of thyroid hormones. Zeitschrift fur Kardiologie 6:219-231, 1996

[28] Novakova D, Uhrova E, Krenek M, Madar J, Tolarova M, Stroufova A: The thyroid gland dysfunction in infertile women. *Am. J. of Reproduct Immunol.* 51:495, 2004

[29] O'Brien T, Dinneen SF, O'Brien PC, Palumbo PJ: Hyperlipidemia in patients with primary and secondary hypothyroidism. *Mayo Clinics Proceedings* 68:860-866, 1993

[30] Papi G, Uberti ED, Betterle C, Carani C, Pearce EN, Braverman LE, Roti E: Subclinical hypothyroidism. *Current Opin. Endocrin. Diabetes Obesity* 14:197-208, 2007

[31] Parle JV, Maisonneuve P, Sheppard MC, Boyle P, Franklyn JA: Prediction of all-cause and cardiovascular mortality in elderly people from one low serum thyreotropin results: a 10-year cohort study. *Lancet* 358:861-865, 2001

[32] Pucci E, Chiovato L, Pinchera A: Thyroid and lipid metabolism. *Int. J. Obes. Metab. Disord.* 24:109-112, 2000

[33] Razvi S, Ingoe L, Keeka G, Oates C, McMillan C, Weaver JU: The beneficial effect of L-thyroxine on cardiovascular risk factors, endothelial function, and quality of life in subclinical hypothyroidism: randomized, crossover trial. *J. Clin. Endocrinol. Metab.* 92:1715-1723, 2007

[34] Rennie JS, MacDonald DG: Quantitative histological analysis of the epithelium of the ventral surface of the hamster tongue in iron deficiency. *Arch Oral Biol.* 1982

[35] Rich AM, Radden BG: Squamous cell carcinoma of the oral mucosa: a review of 244 cases in Australia. *J. Oral Pathol.* 13:459-471, 1984

[36] Schwartz HL, Strait KA, Oppenheimer JH: Molecular mechanisms of thyroid hormone action. A physiologic perspective. *Clinics in Laboratory Medicine* 13:543-561, 1993

[37] Shih A, Lin HY, Davis FB, Davis PJ: Thyroid hormone promotes serine phosphorylation of p53 by mitogen-activated protein kinase. *Biochemistry* 40:2870-2878, 2001

[38] Surks MI, Ortiz E, Daniels GH, Sawin CT, Col NF, Cobin RH, Franklyn JA, Hershman JM, Burman KD, Denke MA, Gorman C, Cooper RS, Weissman NJ: Subclinical thyroid disease: scientific review and guidelines for diagnosis and management. *JAMA* 291:228-238, 2004

[39] Swierczynski J, Mitchell DA, Reinhold DS, Salati LM, Stapleton SR, Klautky SA, Struve, AE, Goodridge AG: Triiodothyronine-induced accumulations of malic enzyme, fatty acid synthase, acetyl-coenzyme A carboxylase, and thier mRNAs are blocked by protein kinase inhibitors. Transcription is the affected step. *J. Biol. Chem.* 266:17459-17466, 1991

[40] Tapia G, Cornejo P, Fernandez V, Videla LA: Protein oxidation in thyroid hormone-induced liver oxidative stress: relation to lipid peroxidation. *Toxicol. Lett.* 106:209-214, 1999

[41] Tsai MJ, O'Malley BW: Molecular mechanisms of action of steroid/thyroid receptor superfamily members. *Anna. Rec. Biochem.* 63:451-486, 1994

[42] Uzunlulu M, Yorulmaz E, Oguz A: Prevalence of subclinical hypothyroidism in patients with metabolic syndrome. *Endocrine J.* 54:71-76, 2007

[43] Velija-Asimi Z, Karamehic J: The effects of treatment of subclinical hypothyroidism on metabolic control and hyperinsulinemia. *Medicinski Arhiv.* 61:20-21, 2007

[44] Walsh JP, Bremner AP, Bulsara MK, O'Leary P, Leedman PJ, Feddema P, Michelangeli V: Thyroid dysfunction and serum lipids: a community-based study. *Clin. Endocrinol.* 63:670-675, 2005

[45] Watts JM: The importance of the Plummer-Vinson syndrome in the aetiology of the upper gastrointestinal tract. *Postgrad. Med. J.* 37:523-533, 1961

[46] Weinstein SP, Watts J, Graves PN, Haber RS: Stimulation of glucose transport by thyroid hormone in ARL 15 cells: increased abundance of glucose transporter protein and messenger ribonucleic acid. *Endocrinology* 126:1421-1429, 1990

[47] Welsch CW: Dietary fat, calories and experimental mammary gland tumorigenesis. *Cancer Res.* 52:2040, 1992

[48] Wiesner RJ, Kurowski TT, Zak R: Regulation by thyroid hormone of nuclear and mitochondrial genes encoding subunits of cytochrome-c oxidase in rat liver and skeletal muscle. *Mol. Endocrinol.* 6:1458-1467, 1992

[49] Winn DM, Ziegler RG, Pickle LW et al: Diet in the etiology of oral and pharyngeal cancer among women from the southern United States. *Cancer Res.* 44:1216-1222, 1984

[50] Wynder EL, Bross IJ, Feldman RM: A study of the etiological factors in cancer of the mouth. *Cancer* 10:1300-1323, 1957

[51] Zhang J, Lazar MA: The mechanism of action of thyroid hormones. *Annu. Rev. Physiol.* 62:439-466, 2000

Epilogue

Conclusions for Cancer Prevention, Cure and Research

Based on the epidemiological experiences and literary data it can be established that smoking associated tumors are not induced only by smoking. Smoking may be regarded as one of many factors that may provoke substantial metabolic and hormonal changes leading to cancer initiation. On the other hand, hormone associated tumors are not induced by estrogen as had been assumed for several decades, rather estrogen loss and the associated insulin resistance are to be blamed for cancer initiation of the highly hormone sensitive organs.

Though cancer initiation is multicausal, estrogen deficiency, either mild or severe, seems to be a crucial factor of carcinogenesis at all sites. Cancer epidemiology of each organ is thoroughly affected by its estrogen sensitivity and estrogen demand. The higher the estrogen demand of an organ the higher the danger of cancer development in an estrogen deficient milieu.

Mild or severe estrogen deficiency is a widespread pathological state both among pre- and postmenopausal women and correction of these hormonal deficiencies supplies many possibilities for cancer prevention. Moreover, balance of the sexual steroid levels may also be crucial for the health of men, but the literary data in this field are relatively scarce.

In otherwise healthy, symptom-free, premenopausal women, mild estrogen deficiency is not only a risk for infertility but also for cardiovascular diseases and cancers. After successful in vitro fertilization and delivery, further strict control of the hormone levels and building up of a regular cycle are advisable to prevent the severe, late complications and fatal outcome of estrogen loss in these women.

In case of women with perimenopausal or postmenopausal complaints hormone therapy is advisable to achieve a symptom-free state and to prevent the late consequences of estrogen deficiency. In cases of unavoidable hysterectomy, at least a one-armed estrogen therapy is advantageous postoperatively even in postmenopausal women, so as to restore the previous individual hormone level of these patients.

A plausible assumption is that cancer induced by estrogen deficiency may be treated by hormone. Estrogen treatment may interfere with local spread and metastatic capacity of cancers both at highly and moderately estrogen sensitive sites. In case of unexpected cancers of young patients, either male or female, a disorder of the equilibrium in male-female sexual steroids and insulin resistance may be supposed. Correction of these hormonal defects may help to cure the malignant processes.

Nowadays, all anticancer agents have severe, toxic effects, killing the hemopoetic cells and thoroughly suppressing the immune system of the patient. One of our old dreams may come true with recognition of the anticancer capacity of estrogen. This new panacea is ideal for cancer cure as it has regulatory effects on cell proliferation and opposes growth factor activities. Moreover, it has beneficial effects on the altered metabolic processes and at the same time is capable of strengthening the immune system.

The theory, which reveals the anticancer capacity of estrogen, may cut a small pathway in the jungle of cancer research. Hopefully, within a few years it will be widened to a highway on which many clinicians and researchers will rush to reach higher levels in prevention and cure of cancer.

Index

A

B

C

D

E

F

I

J

K

L

M

N

O

P

Q

R

T

U

V

W

X

Y